Bonesetters: a History of Osteopathy in Britain

Dedication

The book is dedicated to Anna and Ed who with humour and some fortitude guided me through decades of parenthood.

Bonesetters: a History of Osteopathy in Britain

Author
John C O'Brien MA DO
National Osteopathic Archive, London

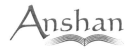

Published by:

Anshan Ltd
11a Little Mount Sion
Tunbridge Wells
Kent. TN1 1YS

Tel: +44 (0) 1892 557767
Fax: +44 (0) 1892 530358

e-mail: info@anshan.co.uk
website: www.anshan.co.uk

ISBN: 978 1 848290 71 6

British Library Cataloguing in Publication Data

A catalogue record for this book is available from the British Library.

Copy Editor: Catherine Lain

Cover Design: Stanley Donwood

Cover Image: Stanley Donwood

Typeset by: Kerrypress Ltd, Luton, Bedfordshire

Printed by:

Contents

About the Author

John O'Brien practised as an osteopath for 40 years. In that time he also taught osteopathic history and clinical studies (although not continuously), including spending 21 years as a final clinical examiner. He gained his MA in the History of Medicine and, recently, has been co-founder and archivist at the National Osteopathic Archive in London.

Introduction

Over the 40 years that I worked as an osteopath I saw great change in the profession. My interest in its history led me to cofound the National Osteopathic Archive (NOA) and it was whilst temporarily storing NOA material in my house that the idea to write this book arose. The size of collected papers and their content fired my enthusiasm. Later, during numerous interviews up and down the country I was impressed by the pride, passion and dedication many osteopaths displayed for their profession.

I could never hope to emulate Martin Collins' broad sweep of British osteopathic history, nor Margery Bloomfield's excellent narrative account of the history of the European School of Osteopathy. However, my research was fortified by many conversations with Martin Collins and Robin Kirk.

Despite my enthusiasm for the subject it would have been easy to become bogged down in peripheral topics and lose direction. I also had to carefully consider how much of the research material should feature, irrespective of its relevance. What gave me some help in pressing ahead was the way that osteopathic history has been handed down in half-truths and superficial generalisations. Historically, this has at times caused friction and wariness among colleagues when a more united profession was attempting to emerge. As Martin has pronounced, a history can fall between two accounts, one readable but lacking scholarship and the other with detailed notation but lacking style and not readily accessible.

The NOA steering committee appeared on occasion to be going round in circles, similar to my literary venture. During a particular period of institutional resistance towards the archive, we were able to draw sustenance from a group of colleagues willing to join an osteopathic history group and meet up four times a year for discussion. In an informal atmosphere of goodwill, these lively symposia produced much debate, devoid of animosity, and perhaps surprisingly so as the history group membership covers a broad spectrum of colleagues from different backgrounds. Their eagerness to understand our history and its relevance furthered my resolve to start the book.

The book's structure emerged when Stephen Tyreman asked me to give a talk to doctoral students about the essential factors influencing osteopathic professional evolution in Britain. This paper became the framework for *Bonesetters*. Each section describes a significant event that enabled the profession to progress and evolve. Each chapter is comprised of three parts. The first gives a brief, informative précis. For those more interested in narrative detail, the second part offers a richer descriptive tapestry. The final section analyses these specific proceedings in order to define them within a reflective context.

The alumni of some colleges will no doubt be apprehensive and perhaps perplexed by my concentration on specific institutions at the expense of their own. Others may feel that certain annals have not been emphasized enough or, perhaps, not even included. My aim is to clarify the past in accessible portions without the reader being overwhelmed by the number of institutions involved or weighed down metaphorically by the complexity of certain situations.

It is possible that some will also be dismayed at the book's title, but it would be wrong to deny osteopathy's origins. Bonesetting has played an important part in the development of osteopathy, chiropractic and modern orthopaedics. There were numerous instances of cooperation between bonesetters and osteopaths during the early decades of the last century. Bonesetters' 'bone out of place' notion and terminology were utilised by AT Still and DD Palmer, founders of osteopathy and chiropractic, respectively. For many years Still advertised himself as the "lightning bonesetter" and J Martin Littlejohn described Still as such a practitioner. For a time, the gifted Sir Herbert Barker, bonesetter extraordinaire, was awarded an honorary doctorate from the American School of Osteopathy, Kirksville, Missouri, and was also appointed a governor of the British School of Osteopathy.

The true heroes of this tale are the early practitioners who dedicated their time and expertise to their communities, often under considerable difficulty. They made it possible for successive generations to enter the by now informed neighbourhoods to practise successfully without duress.

For reasons that can be understood, modern medicine today relies heavily on a considerable armoury of expensive diagnostic aids. A struggling National Health Service provides outstanding results amid limited reserves of time, finance, dedication and unrealised expectations. Despite these and the abilities of alternative practitioners, pandemics of obesity, depression, loneliness, an inability to work and so-called antisocial behaviour continue to gather victims. There are lessons to be learnt from osteopathic history when facing these issues. The usefulness of applying such a method where professionals are trained to decipher these problems, spending time taking detailed case histories including a relevant examination within a biopsychosocial context, is enormously underestimated. This approach is cheap, socially accessible and kind to the environment and its purpose might be of enormous benefit to our communities.

Bonesetters is primarily designed for students as a ready reckoner and one hopes that all those interested in the history of osteopathy will gain something from it. For those seeking a more thorough discourse, it may also act as a launching pad from which to delve further. The book's structure enables practitioners who need to refresh their memory to digest parts of it at leisure or in between gaps in daily practice. Readers will be reminded of the developmental journey osteopathy has taken. At a time when osteopaths appear to be at some crossroad, it is fortuitous, perhaps, to look at our past, learn from it and not re-enact events that have served us ill.

Timeline of Osteopathy in Britain

1898 J Martin Littlejohn gives lecture on osteopathy to members of the Society of Science, Letters and Arts in London.

1902 First osteopaths arrive in UK: Franz Horn in London, Willard Walker in Glasgow and Jay Dunham in Ireland.

1911 US-trained osteopaths form the British Osteopathic Society (in 1916–17 it became the British Osteopathic Association or BOA).

1917 Noel Buxton MP extols the virtues of osteopathy and bonesetting during the 1914–18 war in the House of Commons.
British School of Osteopathy (BSO) set up by J Martin Littlejohn but did not commence until 1922.

1919 Edinburgh School of Natural Therapeutics founded by James Thomson.

1921 William Looker founds the Looker School of Bloodless Medicine (later, the Looker School of Osteopathy and Chiropractic) in Manchester.

1925 BOA unveils its manifesto declaring that manipulation can be confined specifically to themselves and the BSO central to UK education. The British Chiropractic Association, Incorporated Association of Osteopaths (IAO) and Nature Cure Association (legally registered but founded in 1920) were all formed in opposition.
First two BSO students graduate and join the BOA.

1926 Following a successful BOA inspection, J Martin Littlejohn refuses to hand control of the BSO over to an independent BOA Board of Trustees. BOA withdraws all support from the BSO and its alumni, which results in total isolation from its parent American osteopathic institutions.
William Looker dies.

1929 Following the absorption of Looker students and subsequently, students of the British College of Chiropractic/Western School of Osteopathy in Plymouth, BSO alumni join the IAO, consolidating a corps of UK-trained osteopaths.

1935 Select Committee of the House of Lords considers the Registration and Regulation of Osteopaths Bill.

1936 General Council and Register of Osteopaths formed (GCRO).
IAO changes to the Osteopathic Association of Great Britain (OAGB).

1939 BSO gains GCRO accreditation; GCRO assumes OAGB majority and becomes a BSO alumni institution (by 1951 BOA membership on the GCRO has dwindled).

1946 BOA founds the London College of Osteopathy (later, becoming the London College of Osteopathic Medicine) for postgraduate medical training. This coincides with no further US-trained osteopaths arriving to practise in the UK.

1947 J Martin Littlejohn dies.

Shilton Webster-Jones becomes BSO principal. Later, with Clem Middleton, Audrey (née Smith) Lady Percival, Margot Gore and Colin Dove he reappraises the Littlejohn curriculum. Much criticism ensues.

1949 Founding of the British College of Naturopathy (BCN). Stanley Lief is principal.

1951 John Wernham founds the Maidstone Institute of Applied Technique to spread Littlejohn's osteopathy.

1953 The BCN moves to Frazer House, Netherhall Gardens, Hampstead, London.

1961 The BCN changes its name to become the British College of Naturopathy and Osteopathy (BCNO).

1963 Following the Profumo case and involvement of the osteopath, Stephen Ward, the general public becomes aware of osteopathy and its benefits.

Stanley Lief dies.

Albert Rumfitt becomes BCNO principal.

1965 The École Française d'Ostéopathie (EFO) moves to the BCNO.

1966 Demarcation debate between GCRO and OAGB to consider merging. Although 90% have membership of both institutions at this time, the issue creates recriminations that would last decades.

1968 Webster-Jones retires as BSO principal. Colin Dove is appointed principal.

1971 EFO is renamed the École Européene d'Ostéopathie and transfers to Kent.

The Guild of Osteopaths is founded.

1974 European School of Osteopathy founded with Tom Dummer a cofounder and principal. A four year full-time course commences.

1976 Stanley Bradford is appointed BSO principal.

Joyce Butler MP introduces a Bill for the statutory Registration of Osteopaths.

1977 Founding of the Andrew Still College.

1979 ESO moves to its new premises in Tonbridge Road, Maidstone.

The College of Osteopaths Educational Trust (COET) founded.

1980 BSO moves to 1–4 Suffolk Street, Trafalgar Square.

1984 ESO is accredited by the GCRO. Its alumni and members of the Society of Osteopaths join GCRO.

1987 The Croydon School moves to Putney and is renamed the London College of Osteopathy.

1988 The BCNO is GCRO accredited. Its alumni, British Naturopathic and Osteopathic Association join the GCRO.

1989 BSO BSc degree validated.

1991 The King's Fund is set up under Sir Thomas Bingham to review a draft Bill to regulate and register osteopaths.

Margery Bloomfield, cofounder of the ESO, becomes the first woman ESO principal.

The Oxford School is founded.

1992 BCNO awards a BSc in Osteopathic Medicine.

1993 Osteopaths Bill is passed.

The General Osteopathic Council is set up.

The ESO's BSc (Osteopathy) validated and an MSc follows a year later.

1998 LCOM transfers their BOA title for others. The OAGB, BNOA and the Guild join later.

List of Figures

The figures are from the Still Museum of Osteopathic Medicine and the International Center of Osteopathic History, AT Still University, Kirksville, Missouri, USA. The Still Museum has kindly granted imprimatur for the images.

List of Organisations and their Abbreviations

A brief glance through the list of organisations below provides some indication as to the number of individuals that have played a role in one way or another in the development of British osteopathy to date.

AAO   American Applied Academy of Osteopathy
ABO   Association of British Osteopaths
AMA   American Medical Association
AOA   American Osteopathic Association
BAC   British Accreditation Council
BAMM   British Association of Manipulative Medicine
BCA   British Chiropractic Association
BCN   British College of Naturopathy
BCNO   British College of Naturopathy and Osteopathy
BCS   British Chiropractic Society
BOA   British Osteopathic Association
BOS   British Osteopathic Society
BMA   British Medical Association
BNA   British Naturopathic Association
BNOA   British Naturopathic and Osteopathic Association
BSO   British School of Osteopathy
COET   College of Osteopaths
EEO   École Européene d'Ostéopathie
EFO   École Française d'Ostéopathie
ESNT   Edinburgh School of Natural Therapeutics
ESO   European School of Osteopathy
FBCS   Fellow of the British Chiropractic Society
FRCS   Fellow of the Royal College of Surgeons
GCRO   General Council and Register of Osteopaths
GMC   General Medical Council
GOsC   General Osteopathic Council
IAO   Incorporated Association of Osteopaths

IFPNT   International Federation of Practitioners of Natural Therapeutics
LSNT   London School of Natural Therapeutics
OAGB   Osteopathic Association of Great Britain
ODL   Osteopathic Defence League
OGF   Osteopathic Genesis Foundation
OMA   Osteopathic Medical Association
NCA   Nature Cure Association
NOA   National Osteopathic Archive
SCTF   Sutherland Cranial Teaching Foundation
SO   Society of Osteopaths

Acknowledgements

I would like to thank and acknowledge the Still Museum of Osteopathic Medicine and the International Center of Osteopathic History, AT Still University, Kirksville, Missouri for the use of their images in this book. In particular I extend thanks to the director, Jason Haxton, the curator, Debra Loguda-Summers and staff. The Still Museum has kindly granted imprimatur for the images in this book.

I would also like to acknowledge Anne and Sarah Kennard (granddaughter and great granddaughter, respectively) and the National Osteopathic Archive, London.

The early decades of UK osteopathic history present a formidable challenge to anyone attempting to draw up a narrative of those days, precisely because most material was jettisoned periodically from our older institutions and other artifacts were removed surreptitiously over time.

Martin Collins has been solely responsible in saving the remnants of the BSO archive, which happens to be the one of the most valuable collections within the National Osteopathic Archive (NOA). I owe much to Martin, especially his friendship and his scholarship in all matters.[1]

But before taking you along this trail, it should be mentioned how much I owe to certain individuals. Robin Kirk has been a great friend and ally throughout, able to give some refreshing antipodean thoughts. Another antipodean, Margery Bloomfield, has provided her own archive material from the 1950s onwards from the European Schools based in Maidstone. She has given wise and sound counsel with laughter, and is another stalwart NOA trustee. Rachel Martineau has become a good friend and great support throughout. Colin Dove has shown such generosity of spirit in assisting the NOA and extraordinary patience with my lack of ability, at times, to keep up with him. Hilary Beech and her sons opened up an Aladdin's cave of archive material, locked away in the basement of her husband, Gordon's, surgery in Margate for nigh on two decades.

One must not forget an unsung hero from West Country osteopathy, Trenear Michell, who diligently hoarded and catalogued over many decades archive material dating from the 1920s onwards. Anne Pither, Trenear's daughter, stored this material safely. Again, Colin Dove introduced me to Anne, Mich, her brother and her delightful husband, John; Trenear's papers are in safe keeping in our archive.

Among others, Jack Leary generously donated his extensive osteopathic library, containing his father John's, and former British Osteopathic Association (BOA) president, Dora Sutcliffe Lean's. Special mentions go to Garth Robertson, Rod MacDonald, Claude Dutton's family, Max Mitchell-Fox, Robert Lever, Harold Klug, Simon Fielding, Maurice Hills, Marie-Louise Mahieu for her tenacity, Betty Herbert, Lady Audrey Percival, Anne Ellison, Sara Kennard and her mother Anne, and Catherine Goodyear at the BOA. Also at the BSO, I'd like to thank Charles Hunt, Nina Waters, Elizabeth Carter, Jo Smith, Stephen Tyreman, Jorges Estevez, Steve Vogel, Paul Blanchard and Rob McCoy. Many thanks too to all the members of the Osteopathic History Group.

Special thanks to Stanley who took time out from his own art and that of Radiohead to produce such a striking front and back cover. Grateful thanks to Catherine Lain her formidable editing and to my publisher, Andrew White for his valued advice and commitment. My final thanks are to Frank Langan, Anthony Chancellor Weale, Adam Allies, Tom Cree, Nick Harding, my family and to Sue for being there.

References

1.   Collins M., *Osteopathy in Britain*. London: Booksurge. 2005.

Chapter 1

The Rise and Fall of British Bonesetting

Précis

There is little written evidence of bonesetters and their early role in the UK. Nevertheless, certain individuals have stood out over the past four centuries. Early on, bonesetters practised generally in rural areas, their trade being handed down through families and closed groups within such organisations as the Merchant and Royal Navies. They treated both humans and animals, probably as an extension of a rural trade.

Historians have argued that two particular events in the nineteenth century raised the profile of bonesetting and encouraged some medical professionals to take on elements of the craft. The incidents were James Paget's delivery of a lecture entitled 'On the Cases that Bone-setters Cure', published in the British Medical Journal in 1867, and Wharton Hood's treatise 'On Bone-setting' published in 1871. These discourses attempted to persuade colleagues of the merits of the craft and encourage them to acquire these skills for the benefit of their upper and middle class urban/town dwelling patients, and for financial gain as well. Paget and others were only too aware of the impact that homeopathy had had during the second part of the nineteenth century and how successful it had become with these socioeconomic groups.

Bonesetting was in a difficult position. It was seen as a useful discipline to prescribe but many medical practitioners were reluctant to recommend bonesetters because of their lack of education and rudimentary medical training. In addition, the paucity of trade associations and their closed apprenticeships did not help their case. Yet although medical opposition grew, bonesetting did flourish in urban areas and industrial towns and bonesetters maintained practices outside the mainstream medical repertoire.

As bonesetting reached new heights of popularity, so the number of bonesetters increased, much to the chagrin of the medical profession. Bonesetters began to attend vestigial first aid courses to extend their activities to emergency work in factories, football matches and Friendly Society 'sick clubs'. A few bonesetters such as Herbert Barker pursued higher profiles under the dismissive gaze of their medical counterparts, whose professional bodies used their professional clout and legal acumen to discredit Barker.

Bonesetting reached its zenith in the early decades of the twentieth century, practised by crafts people and some medical practitioners. As bonesetting gradually declined, its goodwill, simplistic practice and terminology were utilised by osteopaths, chiropractors and naturopaths. Nevertheless, modern orthopaedics has struggled at times to acknowledge its bonesetting origins.

Historical Examination

The precise origins of bonesetting are unclear[1] but it appears to have evolved from the practises of 'cunning' people such as midwives. Bonesetting was based on a simple biophysical concept which can be defined as a local physical disability or injury that is treated by manual means. Bonesetters used their hands to heal, applying a combination of stroking, rubbing and robust manipulation to provide a 'cure'. It was a naïve unsophisticated craft with a basic 'bone out of place' notion that was based on touch and sight, easy for people to understand and perhaps also hear the possible 'click' elicited from the manipulation. Bonesetting was unbridled by any mysterious, preposterous creed, although some societies believed bonesetters had special gifts for healing. There is little evidence of manipulative techniques being employed in hospitals and yet fracture treatments did become an integral part of general surgery. The craft benefited from a series of remarkable characters, from Valentine Greatrakes in the Restoration period and Sally Mapp in the eighteenth century, to Richard Hutton in the nineteenth century and his relation Sir Herbert Barker in the twentieth century.

It appears that bonesetters never had to compete aggressively for custom. Nor did they organise themselves into coherent political groups, or found bonesetting schools to train their members. Rather, they were closed groups handing down their craft through families or among crew within the Merchant and Royal Navy.[2] Bonesetters had an uncanny knack of moving *out* of areas that the medical profession had begun to consider its own property. For instance, curvatures of the spine such as scoliosis became part of medical practice at the exclusion of bonesetters. As a result, bonesetters moved into *other* areas where the medical profession had no interest. They concentrated instead on common or garden conditions such as aches, sprains and subluxations. It is interesting to note that the general public was able to differentiate those conditions that would require bonesetters' skills from others that needed medical attention and surgical intervention.[3]

Some members of bonesetting families became medical practitioners in their own right including Evan Thomas's three sons, and James Taylor of the Lancashire bonesetting family.[4] Later on these individuals helped to evolve orthopaedics

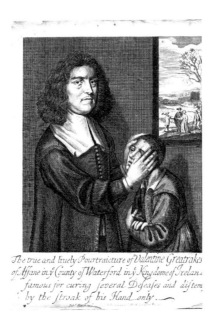

Fig. 1: Valentine Greatrakes

through the absorption of some bonesetting equipment and techniques. The medically qualified Evan Thomas from the famous Welsh family of bonesetters practised his bonesetting skills in Liverpool. Although seen as a guru, Thomas berated bonesetters for their ignorance and hopeless treatment of patients but at the same time castigated medical hierarchy for its apparent pomposity.

Hugh Owen Thomas (Evan's medically qualified son) would have fitted well in early osteopathic ranks, rather than early orthopaedics. He remained resolute, self-sufficient and remote, concentrating on his large practice. It was left to his nephew, Sir Robert Jones, the most prominent pioneer of modern orthopaedics, to impart his uncle's methods to colleagues. Significantly, orthopaedic medicine did not appropriate *all* bonesetting methodology. There remained a modest area of common musculoskeletal and soft tissue conditions among a large proportion of the population for bonesetters to tend.

In 1867 the eminent British surgeon and pathologist Sir James Paget published a paper about bonesetting which identified bonesetters as the enemy and outlined an intended takeover of their medical skill.[5] Paget had been under the tutelage of Sir William Fergusson, a conservative surgeon and advocate of homeopathy. Indeed, many of those surgeons and physicians interested in musculoskeletal

3

medicine were homeopathic supporters too and it had been the one alternative therapy included in Britain's *Medical Act* (1858). Continental Europe and Germany in particular had also embraced Per Ling's medical gymnastics, Vincent Priessnitz's hydrotherapy, massage, and galvanic/electrotherapy. It was after Paget visited Germany that he gave his paper *On the Cases that Bone-setters Cure*, published later in the *British Medical Journal* and subsequently reprinted in 1875 and 1902.

Paget began his lecture with the words: "Few of you are likely to practise without having a bone-setter for an enemy, and if he can cure a case which you have failed to cure, his fortune will be made and yours marred." In that opening gambit Paget vilifies bonesetters as the 'enemy' but paradoxically then goes on to extol bonesetting skills as assets that could be acquired by medical practitioners for the benefit of their upper and middle class clientele, in the process thereby excluding bonesetting's non-medical craftsmen and women. It was quite a turnaround for a medical person to recommend the appropriation of bonesetting skills despite denouncing its therapists.

Meanwhile, it was not unknown for the rich to be treated by traditional bonesetters. For example, Richard Hutton of the Westmorland bonesetting family caused quite a stir among the elite by successfully treating Hon. Spencer Ponsonby of a chronic painful condition when others had failed to do so. Earlier in life Hutton had received medical treatment from Peter Hood and was able to recover from a long and severe bout of illness under Hood's expertise. In gratitude, Hutton promised to teach Wharton Hood, his son, the art of manipulation.[6] Later on, Hutton and Wharton Hood not only treated the poor for free but also imparted the benefits of the craft to upper and middle class Londoners who had already begun to accept the perceived advantages of homeopathy, as advocated by their physicians and surgeons. In time, Sir Robert Jones gathered up much of the bonesetting equipment from Wharton Hood's practice and used his book *On Bone-setting* as a teaching aid to his instruct his orthopaedic students on the salient points of manipulation.[7]

Public awareness of bonesetting grew amid much medical approval and the extolling of virtues of medically acquired skills. Physicians and surgeons did learn manipulative techniques but they were probably taught on an ad hoc basis. As a result an ongoing debate ensued between medical practitioners about whether elements of bonesetting should be integrated into orthopaedic medical practice.[8] Some also extolled the bonesetters' advice of 'getting back to work', a more practical requisite for the working class who were devoid of any sickness benefit.

This was in contrast to the medical middle class professional opinion that rest was the most suitable treatment for physical ailments.

Patients appeared not to distinguish between those who were medically qualified and those who were not, much to the chagrin of the medical professional. Price and the fact that bonesetters were often paid in kind probably added to their popularity. Consequently, more bonesetters began to locate to cities and towns to exploit the demand for their services, much to the annoyance of the medical profession.

In his article 'On Manipulation…as a Means of Surgical Treatment' the surgeon Howard Marsh enquired, "How is it that while herbalists, who hold about the same relationship to medicine that bone-setters hold to surgery, have fallen into the background, bone-setters have rather gained than lost popularity?"[9] What began to vex medical practitioners most was that it was their own approval of bonesetting which had resulted in an increase in bonesetters. The public was quite content to seek out bonesetters regardless of their supposed lack of medical training and their intuitive touch and diligent practice increased further their popularity.[10]

Bonesetting not only survived but also continued to prosper and many bonesetters gained St. John's Ambulance first aid certificates in an effort to broaden their work. Their activities began to extend to factories, Friendly Society 'sick clubs', and sporting activities: places where they did not compete with or threaten orthodox medicine. This facility for moving into areas where medicine had not registered a clinical interest was bolstered, ironically, by the rather humdrum, sheer repetitive nature of the work and the distinct lack of diagnostic skills needed to apply it. Such characteristics were enough to put off any aspiring clinician from taking on their role. Therefore, despite criticism by detractors, bonesetting remained a viable and popular alternative therapy.

It has been argued that in response to bonesetters' rising popularity, the medical profession wanted to use its legal punch to put members of this old craft in their place. Critical gaze focussed on Herbert Barker, bonesetters' de facto leader, a well-known society bonesetter and self-publicist. The upsurge in the fortunes of British bonesetters had coincided with the emergence of their most successful and distinguished practitioner, Sir Herbert Barker. His growing reputation came about because he was not averse at using publicity.[11] However, it also made him a prime target in this conflict with medical authorities.

In 1908, the General Medical Council (GMC) embarked on a series of measures to forestall Barker and his colleagues. Firstly the GMC requested an official parliamentary survey to review "the evil effects produced by the unrestricted practice of medicine and surgery by unqualified persons."[12] Secondly, an aggrieved patient

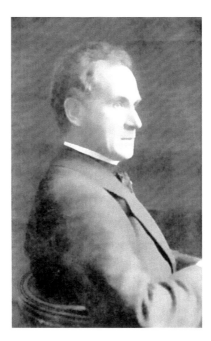

Fig. 2: Herbert Barker

was encouraged to sue Barker through the courts. Although the judge pronounced him guilty, the jury awarded the plaintiff nominal damages. Nonetheless, Barker incurred considerable legal costs and his reputation was tarnished.

The report on unqualified practitioners was published in 1910 and the GMC was proved correct in their assumption. It demonstrated that bonesetters had increased, both in numbers and influence. By 1911, the GMC had decided to thwart bonesetting further by striking off Barker's anaesthetist, Dr WF Axham, from its register, for "infamous conduct".[13] This action backfired on the GMC. The national press, including *The Times*, which normally supported orthodox medicine, described Barker as "having effected perfect cures where regular surgeons had failed."[14] The concerted press campaign had two affects. Firstly, as the GMC was sensitive to hostile opinion no further medical practitioner was penalised for working with bonesetters or osteopaths (although the threat was repeatedly implied over subsequent decades). Secondly, Barker was exonerated and his reputation restored.

These events in the early twentieth century coincided with bonesetting declining as naturopathy, osteopathy and chiropractic gradually began to influence their work and the market. Its demise was characterised by arbitrary training standards and negligible practitioner associations, but its undoubted goodwill and simplified biophysical concepts and terminology were taken on by British osteopathy. While the popularity of bonesetting was on the wane, practitioners of osteopathy, chiropractic and naturopathy began to organise themselves rudimentarily into coherent but distinguishable groups.

Coincidently, a month after the Barker incident on 1st July 1911, The British Osteopathic Society (BOS)[15] became associated with the American Osteopathic Association (AOA). The BOS had been cofounded by Dr Hudson who was "conscious of the strenuous medical opposition" and believed "it was time for (American-trained) osteopaths to form a distinctive organisation."[16] Here was another alternative group, similar to bonesetting, but one that was moving professionally and socially, like Barker, among the establishment in London's West End.

The aspirations of bonesetters and osteopaths overlapped during the First World War. The two groups both made a number of offers to treat wounded soldiers but these were turned down. The excuse given by the War Office was that King's Regulations blocked the employment of any unregistered medical practitioner. However, both groups bypassed this red tape and treated various military personnel privately, many without ever charging a fee. In 1917 this valuable effort was recognised[17] and the first political attempt to overturn "these anomalous conditions" was made through Parliament.[18] Although this failed after the war ended official approval was bestowed on Barker (in 1922 he was knighted for his manipulative services to Royalty and the establishment),[19] and following successful political lobbying, osteopaths were acknowledged as well.[20] Meanwhile, medical authorities repeated dire warnings to those members prepared to work with bonesetters and osteopaths.

Two years later, the GMC reiterated its threat to anaesthetists by cautioning their collaboration with "unregistered persons" and warned that if ignored, it would cause offenders to have their "name erased from the Medical Register".[21] Although this deterred some medical practitioners from assisting bonesetters and osteopaths, others ignored the ruling to continue their association.

The American osteopath Wilfrid Streeter founded the Osteopathic Defence League (ODL) to address this GMC provocation and promote osteopathic political aspirations through influential lay-people support. Sir Herbert Barker, a sympathetic ally, participated in Streeter's ODL. Streeter in return arranged for his alma mater, the American School of Osteopathy, to bestow on Barker an honorary doctorate.[22] Furthermore, a parliamentary friend of Streeter, Arthur Greenwood MP, agreed to question the GMC's discriminatory motives in the House of Commons.[23]

Analysis

As far back as 1656 Robert Turner in *The Compleat Bonesetter* raged against convention, in a vein similar to other reformers and alternative crusaders.[24] Turner's uncompromising position against orthodoxy lives on in osteopathy today, exasperating the healthcare elite and others with protestations and unsubstantiated opinions.

It is possible that the *Medical Act* of 1858 gave medical grandees an opportunity to nail the difference between those medically qualified and the 'great unwashed', in this case, bonesetters. However, in their avarice to extend their areas of influence, Paget and others had actually managed to extol the benefits of bonesetting. The growth of homeopathy and its reputation arising out of Continental Europe played some role in the assimilation of bonesetting within society in the UK. Through the efforts of Sir Robert Jones, some of these pioneering techniques and equipment were introduced into modern orthopaedics.

The GMC and British Medical Association used tactics almost akin to bear-baiting against Sir Herbert Barker, calling off the dogs only after receiving much criticism in the national press about the act of striking Barker's anaesthetist off the Medical Register. No other medical practitioners were struck off for assisting non-medical workers, even though the threat was used on occasion.

When osteopathy made conscious efforts to seek state regulation, medical opponents sought to placate Barker after decades of vilification. He readily acceded to their flattery, distancing himself from osteopaths. Robert Turner and Owen Thomas, on different ends of the spectrum, would have been enraged. By now medical institutions had identified a smaller group, a more lethal 'enemy', and their orthodox spotlight was being fixed on osteopathy.

Bonesetting was assimilated through technique and terminology into osteopathy, chiropractic and nature cure during the early decades of the twentieth century. Indeed, many practitioners used all four titles to describe their practices. Intentionally or otherwise, bonesetting became incorporated into all three. Bonesetting is still practised at one level in the UK and some are registered with Unified Bonesetters Ltd, a non-statutory regulator. It may even be that as it grows as a super power, India, where it is more widely practised, plays a part in a resurgence of bonesetting. Whether it will ever fully emerge as a separate entity again is pure conjecture. However, its proven record stands. Whatever the case, despite the fact that their achievements remain largely unacknowledged, bonesetters can be proud of their past and their continuing influence on chiropractic, orthopaedics, osteopathy and physiotherapy.

References

1. Cooter, R., 'Bones of Contention? Orthodox Medicine and the Mystery of the Bone-Setter's Craft.' Edited by W.F. Bynum & R. Porter, *Medical Fringe and Medical Orthodoxy 1750–1850*. London: Croom Helm. 1981. p.160.
2. Ibid.
3. Dowse, T.S., *Treatment of Disease by Physical Methods*. Bristol: John Wright & Co. 1898. p.255.
4. Collins, M., *Osteopathy in Britain*. London: Booksurge. 2005. p.4.
5. Cooter, pp.167–8.
6. Hood, W., *On Bone-setting*. London: Macmillan & Co. 1871. pp.v–ix.
7. Cooter, pp.168–9.
8. Collins, p.4.
9. Cooter, p.164.
10. Ibid., p.162.
11. Inglis, B., *Natural Medicine*. London: William Collins and Sons. 1979. p.69.
12. Medical Officers of Health to Parliament, *Report as to the Practice of Medicine and Surgery by Unqualified Persons in the United Kingdom*. 1910.
13. Collins, p.8.
14. Barker H.A., *Leaves from My Life*. London: Hutchinson & Co. 1927. p.124.
15. British Osteopathic Association, *Osteopathy in Wartime*. 1943. p.5.
16. Booth, E.R., *History of Osteopathy*. Cincinnati: Caxton Press. 1924. p.652.
17. NOA LCOM/Miscellaneous/File 1. *Speech by Noel Buxton MP*. House of Commons 14th August 1917. pp.1–3.
18. British Osteopathic Association, *Osteopathy in Wartime*. 1943. pp.15–16.
19. BMA, Medico-political Committee minutes June 6 1917. p.683. Item 120.
20. Inglis, pp.73–4.
21. Collins, p.49.
22. British School of Osteopathy, *Prospectus*. 1927–8.
23. Collins, p.51.
24. Cooter, p.165.

Chapter 2

The Establishment of Osteopathy in Britain

Précis

This chapter concentrates on osteopathic training facilities and the establishment of its associations during osteopathy's formative years in the early twentieth century. In the first decade of the twentieth century graduates from US osteopathic colleges started to arrive in the UK in small numbers. J Martin Littlejohn marked two visits to Britain with talks on osteopathy. It took 20 years for the number of osteopaths to increase and by then the profession included a group of British practitioners whose training had varied. Osteopathy comprised of graduates from US colleges allied to the American Osteopathic Association (AOA), US graduates from non-affiliated AOA colleges, those from UK training establishments and others apprenticed to osteopaths, some taking correspondence courses and yet more self-taught from manuals. They advertised themselves variously as bonesetters, chiropractors, naturopaths and osteopaths, a practice that continued for subsequent decades.

The earliest recorded osteopathic organisation comes from the US. AOA allied but not affiliated graduates formed the British Osteopathic Society (BOS) in 1911. It has been established that the BOS was still in existence in 1915 and sometime between then and 1923 it metamorphosed into the British Osteopathic Association, adding ten further members to its BOS directory of 26 practitioners. JM Littlejohn had spoken on a number of occasions with others about founding the British School of Osteopathy. It has never been established whether he had set up a rudimentary school in 1917, but we do know that the first two students graduated in 1925.

William Looker established his own school in Manchester in 1921. Looker had graduated from an assortment of US colleges in naturopathy, chiropractic and osteopathy. He returned to Britain to practise osteopathy and so-called bloodless surgery. One of the Manchester school's alumni was Tom Mitchell-Fox, who later became Dean of the British College of Chiropractic. The College was established in London 1925 and transferred to Plymouth two years later. In 1928 Mitchell-Fox founded the Western Osteopathic School in the same building in Plymouth. All three schools were absorbed, directly or indirectly, into the British School of Osteopathy.

JM Littlejohn's custom of giving students credits for previous training __not__ undertaken at other establishments had serious repercussions. During the Select Committee hearings at the House of Lords Osteopaths Bill (1935) JM Littlejohn and the BSO were vilified. Further associations were founded including the Incorporated Association of Osteopaths (IAO) in 1925 and the Association of British Osteopaths (ABO) in 1926 for British School of Osteopathy (BSO) alumni. The ABO was subsumed into the IAO, three years later. Although the IAO became the largest group of British-trained osteopaths, it was the numerically smaller BOA, who appeared to have become the most influential.

Historical Examination

In 1898, 1899 and 1903, J Martin Littlejohn, a Glaswegian who had learnt the practise of osteopathy under the father of osteopathy himself, AT Still, visited London to give talks introducing the benefits of osteopathy to middle class audiences. History now sees him as the man who brought osteopathy to the UK.

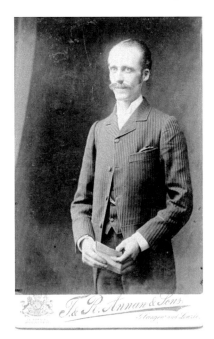

Fig. 3: JM Littlejohn, 1890

The last visit provided a meeting with L Willard Walker and Franz Horn, both recent osteopathic arrivals to the UK. They had been preceded a year before by

Jay Dunham who had become the first osteopath in the UK, practising in Belfast and Dublin.[1] As described in Chapter 1, we know that from 1908, the General Medical Council (GMC) had earmarked the society bonesetter, Herbert Barker, for hostile pursuit through the law courts. Around the same time the GMC began its petition for a parliamentary enquiry into unregistered practitioners, which later reported a growth in the number of bonesetters. Subsequently the press reported an unfair GMC vendetta against Barker and his anaesthetist, striking the latter off the medical register. The British Osteopathic Society (BOS) was founded in 1911 against this backdrop of GMC vindictiveness.[2]

Details of the exact date that the BOS originated and its metamorphosis into the British Osteopathic Association (BOA) are unclear. We know the BOS continued to exist as an authoritative group for American-trained osteopaths and was allied to the American Osteopathic Association but significantly it was not subordinated to them. In fact, we do know the BOS existed up to and including 1915. Its directory contained 26 members throughout the UK, of which 11 were women and 16 of whom worked in central London.[3] Some think that one of them, Georgiana Watson practising in London, was the first female osteopath. Others venture that Marion Hall practising in Glasgow and later in London has that accolade. Dr Franklyn Hudson, practising in Edinburgh, supervised its foundation meeting at the Midland Hotel in Manchester. His was a clarion call for US graduates to gather under the BOS heading as a "collective and distinct organisation". The earliest surviving BOA directory is undated; the BOA came into being sometime between 1915 and 1923.[4]

A MANIFESTO

from

The British Osteopathic Association

THE BRITISH OSTEOPATHIC ASSOCIATION is an Association of fully trained and qualified practitioners of Osteopathy.

I.   Osteopathy is that system of the art of healing which regards the structural integrity of the body as the most important single factor in the maintenance of health. It relies upon the manual removal of framework abnormalities for the restoration of health. It is recognised by the laws of the 48 States of the United States of America and of certain provinces of the Dominion of Canada.

II.   Because of their qualifications, the Members of the Association have been granted full legal recognition in these countries, and their training has been received at one or other of the ASSOCIATED COLLEGES OF OSTEOPATHY approved by the American Osteopathic Association. Many of the Members are British-born men and women, who have been compelled to go to the United States of America to receive their training and to become qualified Osteopaths. The Association has recognised with pleasure the work of Sir Herbert Barker.

Fig. 4: BOA Manifesto

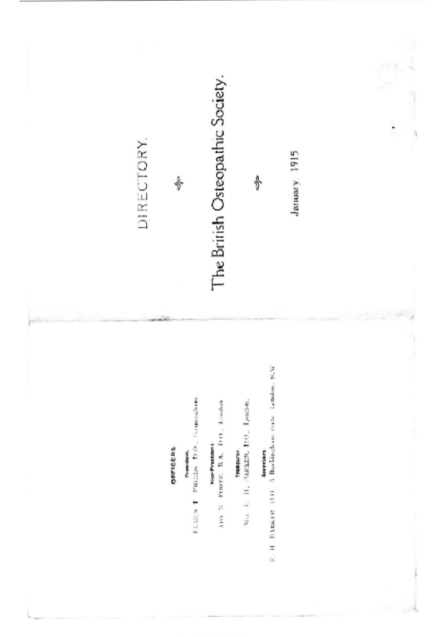

Fig. 5: BOS Directory

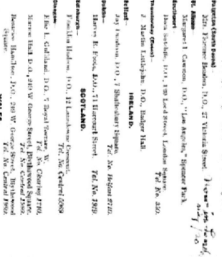

Fig. 6: BOS Membership 1915

By 1923–4 the BOA had grown to include 36 members, 11 of whom were women. At this time 26 practitioners were working in central London. Elmer Pheils, one time BOS president and BOA vice-president, wrote an article entitled 'Osteopathic Propaganda in England' published in the *Journal of the AOA*, which cited grievances against medical action towards osteopaths.

Repeated attempts were made during the First World War for official approval to be given to osteopaths to treat war casualties. In a speech on 14 August 1917 the MP Noel Buxton stated:

"The value of Bonesetters and Osteopaths is admitted. The Government know it quite well. The numbers of discharged men are now, of course, enormous …Clearly a large number of those cases discharged now as incurable are susceptible to treatment, and if a method of cure is being neglected it really is an extremely serious matter, and I think the obstacle to the use of such a method is one which should be removed."[5]

However, such propositions were met by relentless medical opposition. Pheils continued to bewail the misappropriation of osteopathic procedures by orthopaedists, although there were some exceptions.[6]

One highly influential early osteopath was William Looker. In his youth he had displayed much musical talent, like many osteopaths after him. At just 18 years old he was already a talented organist and choirmaster for a number of churches in the Warrington and Manchester district. At the same time he ran and conducted a number of male voice choirs and choral societies. These groups included medical practitioners who may have fuelled his interest in medical matters.

In 1909 Looker registered as a student at the American College of Mechanotherapy, Philadelphia, a city with good institutions for medical and paramedical training. He spent two years as a mechano-therapist and then attended the American School of Naturopathy, New York City, where he came under the influence of one of the greatest nineteenth century naturopaths, Benedict Lust. Looker enrolled at the National College of Chiropractic, Grand Rapids, Michigan in 1913. The following year he purportedly sat his final exams in medicine and surgery. It is thought that two years on he trained under Charles Murray at the International College of Osteopathy, Elgin, a non-AOA affiliated establishment. We can only speculate at the quality of these various institutions. As rumour has it, he had to leave America in a hurry and return to England.[7]

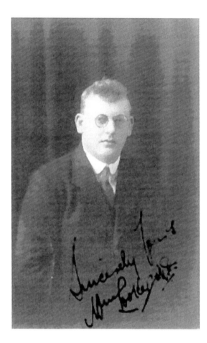

Fig. 7: William Looker

Looker founded The Manchester School of Osteopathy and Bloodless Surgery in 1921, later shortening its title to the Manchester School of Osteopathy. In his writings Looker extolled the virtues of AT Still who he believed "developed this wonderful science [although] he had no intention that Osteopaths should presume to be medical physicians and surgeons ...It took the place entirely as a method treatment, after he had developed, of his medical and surgical methods."[8]

Looker castigated some osteopathic schools for mirroring orthodox schools, when 18 month to 2 year courses were sufficient to train traditional practitioners. He presupposed, "Osteopathy includes all methods of drugless healing, *but it does, and never did, include medication in the form of drugs, and its principles cannot be changed from the lines of practice as laid down by its noble founder"* (his italics). He berates those osteopaths who prescribe drugs, anaesthetise and perform major surgery in the same way as a medical physician and surgeon.[9] Looker reflected osteopathic traditional views as opposed to those osteopaths, more resolute after Still's death, who advocated Abraham Flexner's North American medical school reforms which orthodox medicine was going through. Two years on, Looker had changed his school's name again and his views reflected a more critical understanding of Still's traditional osteopathy.

In 1923 the school was renamed The Looker College of Osteopathy and Chiropractic.[10] This change had arisen from Looker's reappraisal of his interpretation of both osteopathy and chiropractic. From his perspective, Looker was unaware that AT Still had practised for the best part of two decades as the 'lightning bonesetter'. He draws on evidence from Bohemia and Germany where "the patient would lie on upon the floor while another walked on his back, one foot being placed on either side of the spinous process" and the Indians, describing "the patient being tied to a tree and his back being then vigorously pounded".

According to Looker, the Bohemians were the first to employ the 'definite thrust' but were not trained in 'spinal analysis'. He appears to conclude that the pedigree of the founder of chiropractic, DD Palmer, is directly related to those early natural healers and the development of the chiropractic thrust arose from these origins. However, he criticised both Still and Palmer, stating "there is no question that the progress of both of these sciences (osteopathy and chiropractic) was much delayed by the contentions of these pioneers. We well know, with our knowledge of Pathology, that such views could not be subscribed to by anyone who had a liberal training ...Palmer apparently did not understand Pathology".[11] Yet neither did Still and many of his Kirksville faculty who found fault in its advocacy by the Littlejohn brothers and Bill Smith, who were all instantly dismissed from the faculty (although the Littlejohns at least were allowed to finish their training).[12] Looker remained a restless person, transferring with his wife, Rosanna, his home and practice to London.

Looker's title was 'Osteopathic Surgeon' and he practised at 54 Elm Park Gardens, London SW 10, between the Fulham and Kings Road, Chelsea. On the morning of 27th July 1926, following a chill caught a week previously, Looker died from pneumonia, aged 44 years. Two months later, *Health and Efficiency* published his obituary, eulogising a man cut short in his prime. Looker evoked considerable enthusiasm for his duality of chiropractic and osteopathy.

William Looker was a consistent fellow, controversial in both life and death. Following his passing, Rosanna sued Law Union and the Rock Insurance Company for £5,000.00 after they refused to pay out on a recently purchased policy. The judge, Mr Justice Acton, ruled in the company's favour, stating that the policy had been invalid because they had been unaware of his change in health. In one step Rosanna not only lost her husband but also her money.[13]

Under the auspices of Chairman Ernest Davies, 14 founder members of the IOA met at Milton Hall in Manchester on 30th May 1925. It was agreed that "all Looker college students should be given sympathetic consideration and (IAO) existence, should they appeal to the association."[14] Although the IAO showed a degree of approval towards Looker alumni, William Looker was never directly involved in its organisation; he had already formed the British Association of Osteopathy (Incorporated).[15] Whether this was a forerunner of the IAO would only be supposition. However, we do know that after his death a year later, the Association felt hamstrung when the college was wound up. Mr RA Buck of Rochdale appealed to the IAO council for assistance "as he had paid full fees but had not graduated". Indeed, many students beseeched the council in similar circumstances; its response was to negate any responsibility for their plight.

In the north of England, 99% of Looker graduates, nicknamed Lookercytes, formed another osteopathic group, the Incorporated Association of Osteopaths (IAO),[16] although a few Lookercytes became members of a transient group, the National Osteopathic Association of the United Kingdom.[17]

It was JM Littlejohn who came to the rescue and arranged for these students to graduate at the BSO. There were a dozen Looker students under JM Littlejohn's tutelage, all based in Lancashire and who travelled down to London one weekend in four. Benefitting from JM Littlejohn's personal direction and assessment, these 12 students went on to gain their BSO diplomas and became a crucial northern core of osteopathy for many decades.[18]

The IAO was also involved in arranging examinations for aspiring graduate members, organising postgraduate talks and opening clinics in Manchester and Liverpool, the latter run by a bonesetter, Mr Kenwood. Meanwhile, Ernest Davies, President of the National School of Naturopathy, gave details of the college and his correspondence with Benedict Lust. Arthur Millwood gave a critique on the works of Joy Loban, an outstanding chiropractor who had marched, together with many students, out of the college of the outstanding entrepreneur and chiropractor BJ Palmer (son of DD Palmer) in Davenport to found his own down the street. JM Littlejohn's help with Looker students led an IAO delegation to meet up with him in London. In 1929, the BSO alumni, the Association of British Osteopaths (ABO), were subsumed into the IAO.[19]

The British Chiropractic College was established in 1925 at Taviton Street, off Euston Square, London EC1. Its dean was A Warde Allen. The college transferred to Plymouth two years later, Allen having relinquished his position as principal to the Glaswegian Tom Mitchell-Fox, an ex-army physical instructor who shared and adhered to Looker's philosophy. Its alumni joined the British Chiropractic Society (BCS) and their members were permitted to use the suffix FBCS (Fellow of the British Chiropractic Society), which is not dissimilar to FRCS (Fellow of the Royal

College of Surgeons). Most of these practitioners used a combination of osteopathy, chiropractic, naturopathy and some bonesetting. In comparison, the British Chiropractic Association (BCA) founded in 1925 just accepted American-trained 'straight' (only chiropractic) members.

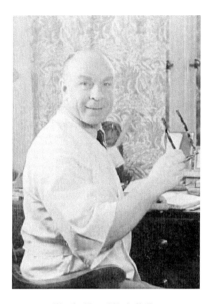

Fig. 8: Tom Mitchell-Fox

Mitchell-Fox decided to found an osteopathic sister college in the same building as the British Chiropractic College at 6 Leigham Street, The Hoe, Plymouth. The Western School of Osteopathy opened its doors for students on the 6th September 1928.[20] How long it lasted and the number of students who attended is unknown. We do know that both establishments existed up to April 1929 although Mitchell-Fox had left his wife for his secretary the year before. His ex-wife's family had been substantial in his private and professional life. Trenear Michell, his brother-in-law, had graduated in the previous summer from the British Chiropractic College and worked as an assistant in Mitchell-Fox's practice. His former mother-in-law had given him space in her home to develop his practice in Plymouth. Estranged from his wife and her family, it is alleged that Mitchell-Fox dismissed his brother-in-law from his practice and Mitchell-Fox's schools foundered, their infrastructure too fragile to continue. A few students attending transferred to the BSO and JM Littlejohn continued his dubious arrangement of crediting 'Lookercytes' with work they had not completed at their former establishment. In the case of one former Plymouth student, a BSO diploma was issued without the student having to do any further study.[21]

Analysis

The early decades of the twentieth century were critical for osteopathy. It could not develop its professionalism through legislation for a number of reasons. American osteopathy's evolution was due to mid-Western state legislation, areas where states were evolving their legislature during their formative decades. There was no opportunity for British osteopathy to achieve similar success though Parliament because medical opposition was so strong. There were few osteopaths and these were located in smallish concentrations. A few American osteopaths did practise in Britain, with the majority working in central London.

Looker's school based in Manchester gave rise to the Incorporated Association of Osteopaths. Its 14 founder members were mostly situated in Lancashire. From this core came Willis Haycock, Pat Saul, Arthur Millward and John Leary, all bastions of northern osteopathy. Looker meanwhile had moved south to London and perhaps the school might have transferred too if he had not died so abruptly.

JM Littlejohn welcomed the twelve Looker students, "the apostles", to finish their training at the BSO in a circumscribed fashion. He gave them all credits for training which none had undertaken at Manchester and their BSO examinations were very rudimentary to say the least.

When the British Chiropractic College and vestigial Western School of Osteopathy collapsed in Plymouth due to Mitchell-Fox's personal problems, several students agreed to JM Littlejohn's terms at the BSO. Unfortunately, JM Littlejohn's behaviour during these events subsequently led the Select Committee for the Osteopaths Bill, House of Lords to report, "the school was of negligible importance and in thoroughly dishonest hands". For all JM Littlejohn's undoubted ability, it put osteopathic legislation back 60 years. But JM Littlejohn's personal commitment to his BSO meant that he could still rely on some of its alumni to assist him in the running of the school. The Looker school and Plymouth establishments folded due to fragile infrastructures.

The trickle of American osteopaths arriving in Britain had virtually ceased by 1940. Unlike some organisations, the IAO was not completely London-orientated, having its Lancashire and south western regions from Looker and Plymouth alumni to develop a better spread of practitioners. These pioneers worked long hours for many decades, sometimes doing six days per week. Their dedication,

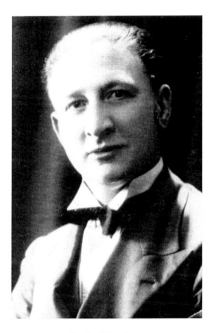

Fig. 9: John Leary

with little help outside their numbers, meant that they became valuable practitioners establishing practices within their communities. Such foundations led to successive osteopathic generations entering towns that were familiar with the practise of osteopathy.

References

1. General Council and Register of Osteopaths, *The Osteopathic Blue Book: the origin and development of osteopathy in Great Britain*. London: GCRO. 1957. pp.9–11.
2. Booth, E.R., *History of Osteopathy*. Cincinnati: Caxton Press. 1905. p.652.
3. NOA Tom Mitchell-Fox Archive. *The British Osteopathic Society Directory*. January 1915.
4. NOA Tom Mitchell-Fox Archive. *The British Osteopathic Association*. (Undated).
5. NOA LCOM/Miscellaneous/File 1. *Speech by Noel Buxton MP*. House of Commons 14th August 1917. pp.1–3.
6. Booth, p.652.
7. Spencer, G., NOA/Early Ost./Chiro. Schools/Vol. 1.
8. Looker, W 'What Osteopathy is Not.' *Health and Efficiency*. 1921–2 (?). NOA/Early Ost./Chiro. Schools/Vol. 1.
9. Ibid.

10. NOA/Early Ost/Chiro. Schools/Vol.1. *Health and Efficiency*. June 1923. p.297.

11. Looker, W., 'The Origin of Chiropractic.' *Health and Efficiency*. June 1923. p.280. NOA/Early Ost./Chiro. Schools/Vol.1.

12. Hildreth, A.G., *The Lengthening Shadow of Andrew Taylor Still*. Kirksville: Journal Printing. 1938. p.124.

13. £5,000 Insurance Policy – widow's claim fails. *Daily Mail* (undated). NOA/Early Ost./Chiro. Schools/Vol.1.

14. NOA/IAO/AGM/Council Meetings 30/05/1925–12/12/1942 p.1.

15. Floyd McKeon, L.C., *Osteopathy and Chiropractic Explained*. London: Lutterworth's. 1927. p.32.

16. Floyd McKeon, L.C., *Health and Efficiency*. Dec 1928. p.626. NOA/Early Ost. /Chiro. Schools/Vol. 1.

17. Spencer, G., *The Looker College of Osteopathy and Chiropractic and its Founder*. NOA/Early Ost./Chiro. Schools/Vol.

18. Leary, Jack., NOA/DVD Interview. 2008.

19. NOA/IAO/AGM/Council Meetings 1925–42. pp.15–17.

20. NOA/Early Ost./Chiro. Schools/Vol.1. *Western Osteopathic School*. Handwritten preliminary announcement.

21. NOA/J. Martin Littlejohn Archive. Littlejohn personal letters to Trenear Michell and his mother explaining the doubtful diploma.

Chapter 3

A Parting of the Ways: the Split of British and American Osteopathy in 1926

Précis

The first decade of the twentieth century brought forth traumatic and irrevocable events in American osteopathy which would resonate again in 1926 in the UK. During this period it is useful to consider J Martin (JM) Littlejohn's relationship with his brothers William, James and David, with Andrew Taylor Still and also his abandonment of life in Chicago for Britain, where he returned to live with his young family.

Still claimed that he had been given osteopathy as a gift from the Almighty. In order to support that pronouncement he carefully obscured his past. However, there is ample evidence to show that Still gleaned many of his ideas from alternative medical sources and his apparent originality is to be found in his assembly of them.

JM Littlejohn was aware of some of Still's influences and his early osteopathic writings were unwittingly far superior. Conflict among the Littlejohn brothers and fellow Scot, Bill Smith, and the remaining Kirksville faculty members over some trumped up charges resulted in Still sacking them all, but the Littlejohns were allowed to finish their course. The three brothers cofounded and ran the Chicago Osteopathic College for over a decade. As the eldest of the three and assuming his intellect was the greater, JM Littlejohn took the helm. However, the partnership ended in 1912 when James, who was actually a far better lecturer, and a delegation of Chicago osteopaths dispossessed JM Littlejohn of that role. The brothers had to accede to an independent board of trustees controlling the college. At the heart of the crisis, JM Littlejohn could not maintain his Chicago colleagues' support for his more expansive concept. Instead they wished to endorse a traditional osteopathic course.

Feeling betrayed by his colleagues and his brothers, JM Littlejohn returned to Britain with his wife Mabel and six young children. He was able to purchase outright Badger Hall in Essex and also a long lease on a Mayfair flat from co-ownership of the Chicago College, academic posts and practice. He founded the British School of Osteopathy (BSO) in 1917 although its first students did not graduate until 1925.

25

The British Osteopathic Association (BOA) wanted ownership of the BSO to be handed over to an independent board of trustees too. This time JM Littlejohn was adamant and he refused. As a result, the BOA, an honorary associate institution of the American Osteopathic Association (AOA), cut all ties.

In time, JM Littlejohn assisted other British osteopathic schools and associations to unite under a single school, the BSO and one association, The Incorporated Association of Osteopaths (IAO). All official contact between British-trained osteopaths and their American parent organisation the AOA was abandoned and their destinies separated.

Historical Examination

During the turn of the nineteenth and twentieth century, faculty members of the American School of Osteopathy (ASO) Kirksville, William Smith and the three Littlejohn brothers (excluding William), were verbally accosted by other faculty associates.

Opposition was headed by AG Hildreth, W Laughlin and Carl McConnell, who led a delegation of disaffected colleagues to Still to voice their protestations against medical subjects having preference in the curriculum over osteopathic ones; and a supposed academic arrogance of the Smith and the Littlejohns towards their fellow faculty colleagues. It was declared that unless this situation was addressed by Still then these majority faculty members would resign en masse. Allegedly many students appeared to reflect this view. Faced with such opposition Bill Smith resigned instantly. The Littlejohn brothers were allowed to complete their studies and then moved on to Chicago.[1]

This episode illustrates a paradox facing early osteopathy, the issue of maintaining a balance between the theoretical knowledge offered by academia and the practical manual skills required by practitioners. Still rather relished his public persona as the Abe Lincoln of medical opposition, his character was easily understood by others yet his shrewd guile was well disguised.[2] He was a complex, intelligent autodidact, mistrustful of the scholarly attributes in some of his staff and discouraging of those prepared to evolve his ideas or interpret his principles in such a way that might give them credence over him.

We do not know whether Still was orchestrating the situation at the ASO to his advantage in order to scupper any rival claim to his mantle. Still could have viewed any notable academic contribution with suspicion but JM Littlejohn was a true academic who appeared to understand Still's concepts, much to the founder's chagrin. Smith and the Littlejohn brothers were simply endeavouring to raise the pretty basic standards among many students (and perhaps even some staff) whose

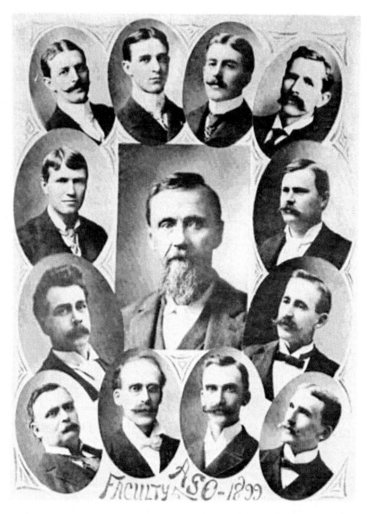

W. R. Laughlin	M. E. Clark	Carl P. McConnell	H. J. Still
Charles Still			H. M. Still
	A. T. STILL (centre)		
William Smith			D. H. Hildreth
Judge Andrew Ellison	J. M. Littlejohn	J. B. Littlejohn	David Littlejohn

Fig. 10: ASO Faculty 1899

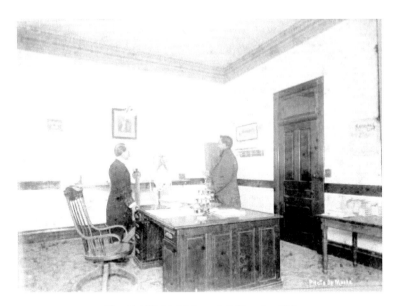

Fig. 11: *JM Littlejohn and Still at the ASO*

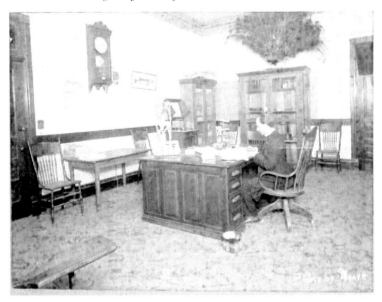

Fig. 12: *JM Littlejohn at Kirksville 1898–1900*

education was limited. The incident was a precursor to future skirmishes and battles among traditionalists and reformers, which would continue in the USA until the early 1960s and result in the eventual capitulation of traditionalists.

It is known that all three brothers cofounded the American College of Osteopathic Medicine and Surgery in Chicago in 1900. JM Littlejohn became its president from the inauguration.[3] Subsequently, the College absorbed the Chicago School of Osteopathy and by 1909 it had been renamed the Littlejohn College of Osteopathy.[4]

However, challenges lay ahead. Flexner's *Report on Medical Education in America and Canada* published in 1910 stated that a basic requirement for all medical schools, including osteopathic ones, was the appointment of an independent board of trustees. Two years later, an independent board of trustees at Chicago was ratified taking financial control away from the Littlejohn brothers. Even more significantly, the presidency was withdrawn from JM Littlejohn. This was implemented by a delegation of Chicago osteopaths headed by Carl McConnell and James Littlejohn, who had masterminded a plan to refuse to ratify JM Littlejohn as head. JM Littlejohn felt doubly betrayed by McConnell who had been one of the ringleaders in ousting the three brothers and Smith from Kirksville a decade before. Even worse, as far as JM Littlejohn was concerned, was to suffer as he had at the hands of his co-conspiring brothers, James and to a lesser extent, David.

The family discord led to an irreconcilable rift which never healed between JM Littlejohn and his two brothers. Like James, their eldest brother, William, had qualified in medicine in Glasgow. We do know that William emigrated to the USA but he had resolutely any ignored osteopathic inclinations. Whether he had influenced his two brothers to moderate their views on it would be conjecture, but James and David never communicated again with JM Littlejohn after this debacle. James went on to become president of the newly created Chicago College of Osteopathy. He became an early reformer of what is referred to as three-fingered rather than ten-fingered osteopathy – a reference to the three fingers required to give an injection.[5] James was instrumental, among others, in guiding osteopathic development towards surgery and implementation of the *Materia Medica,* which was unsuccessful in 1909 but *was* introduced into all American Osteopathic Association (AOA) accredited schools twenty years later. JM Littlejohn was somewhat dismissive of this form of practice. His exile to Britain was a terrible loss to his leaderless reforming colleagues, who were hesitant to return to basic manipulative practice as expressed by the majority. A growing minority began to push for full pharmacological and surgical rights. David meanwhile had moved away from osteopathy to become a thrice-married officer of public health and sanitation.[6]

JM Littlejohn continued to develop his ideas in a steadfast way, pursuing his academic and professional career, teaching and writing, during the first decade of the twentieth century. He had understood much of Still's ideas and related them to those beyond the 'bone out of place' concept causing illness. His academic qualities, unappreciated by some at ASO, Kirksville, had found credence in Chicago.

After Flexner's report things began to change rapidly in medical education. The next twenty-five years saw a complete orthodox medical implementation of Flexner's proposals. In 1935, American Osteopathic Association schools took Flexner reforms on board and these were completed by 1960.[7] A lack of academic content had weighed heavily against the traditionalists, especially after Still's death in 1917. Moreover, the loss of an academic achiever like JM Littlejohn to counter faith, loyalty and dogma[8] as osteopathic prerequisites for US traditionalists, continued to create divisions within the profession. Yet these factors were not enough to sustain a minority cohort of practitioners who were leading the profession away from Still's shadow. These reforming osteopaths found recompense in distancing themselves from traditionalists and felt a greater affinity towards orthodox medicine, encouraged too by the discovery of synthetic drugs such as Salvarsan[9] and later, sulphonamides, penicillin and streptomycin.[10]

JM Littlejohn's tragedy was that he was unable to encourage those traditionalists prepared to share his grander vision. In 1913 he took his wife Mabel and six young children back to Britain, but he no longer had a large stage from which to conduct his message. Events had left him feeling humiliated and betrayed and further fallout came to haunt him yet again twelve years later.

In 1925 the British Osteopathic Association (BOA), the professional body of the American Osteopathic Association (AOA) accredited graduates, gave its support to JM Littlejohn's British School of Osteopathy (BSO) and encouraged 11 members to join the BSO faculty.[11] The school trained undergraduates over a four-year period and medical graduates during a year-long course. At the same time, the first two BSO graduates, Elsie Wareing and Gerald Lowry, were allowed membership to the BOA.

In early 1926,[12] JM Littlejohn, President of the BOA but also Dean of the BSO, met a BOA delegation to transfer control of the school to an independent board of trustees, similar to other AOA accredited schools and according to Flexner's basic requirements for evolving medical education. Yet JM Littlejohn's steadfastness could turn into downright obstinacy if he didn't take to individuals[13] and he was not prepared to hand his BSO over to any board. The shadow of fratricidal struggles and loss of his pivotal role at the Chicago College cast a bleak shadow over these events.

JM Littlejohn had identified the BSO as a steady form of income: student fees and payments from patients attending BSO student clinics. Be that as it may, he was left in no doubt that failure to give into the demands would lead to BOA withdrawal of BSO accreditation and support, leaving it totally isolated from its AOA parent organisation. A final attempt was made by the BOA in September 1926 to persuade JM Littlejohn to transfer the school to a BOA board of trustees. He was made aware once again of the implications of failure that would result in enforced separation from the AOA. His continued intransigence resulted in the BOA's departure from the BSO. Apart from Dr Martisus and Dr Harvey Foote who joined the new faculty, no other BSO graduates joined the BOA and the AOA abandoned accreditation. JM Littlejohn did resign as president and his membership of the BOA in response to these actions.

Meanwhile, William Looker had died unexpectedly a month earlier. Students and graduates of his School of Bloodless Surgery in Manchester (later called the Looker College of Osteopathy and Chiropractic), went to the Incorporated Association of Osteopaths (IAO) asking for assistance to finish the courses that had been abruptly terminated by Looker's death. The IAO had been formed by a number of Looker graduates a year before. They were unable to provide help for the students affected but someone suggested approaching JM Littlejohn. He did duly help these twelve students, calling them 'the apostles' and enabling them to complete their training under the auspices of the BSO in a year. He gave them three year's credit for study at the Looker school even though some critics believed the Looker course to be less than six months long. Looker graduates and members of the IAO were assimilated too as BSO graduates.[14]

In July 1927, IAO members agreed to submit to a year's study supervised by a member of the BSO faculty through viva voce and 'clinical demonstrations', although they refused to countenance written exams because it was thought that "by so doing, their position as a corporation was being forfeited". Whatever this inferred, it did mean that the IAO members respected JM Littlejohn's views on upgrading their skills and they were prepared to concede to a year's study and some form of viva and clinical examination at the end in order to gain their BSO diplomas. However, JM Littlejohn had to compromise rather too much by yielding the necessary requirement to sit written exams.[15] The concession of lowering standards for BSO diplomats and the three year dispensation for Looker students would come back to haunt him in the House of Lords Select Committee sessions in 1935.

By 1929, JM Littlejohn's BSO graduate association, the Association of British Osteopaths, had become absorbed into the IAO. Students and graduates of the Western School of Osteopathy and British Chiropractic College were awarded BSO diplomas and were able to join its professional association, the IAO. Having been isolated from their AOA parent, JM Littlejohn rallied disparate groups of British-trained osteopaths, chiropractors and naturopaths under the BSO fiefdom. He displayed relentless energy at this time, running the BSO, continuing to practise in London and providing for his large family in Thundersley, Essex. His audience was small but appreciative and they appeared to admire his leadership. To them he gave his own interpretation of Still's concepts, even though it left many baffled. However, he had jettisoned one of his vital ideas of human adjustment and adaption which he formulated during his tenure at Chicago, probably his greatest hypothesis.

Eventually the separation between the BOA and the BSO/IAO practitioners became unbridgeable, even when both sides were encouraged to cooperate. An amalgam of osteopaths, chiropractors and naturopaths came together within the IAO under JM Littlejohn's tutelage to evolve British osteopathy, independent of the AOA, and expand it throughout Europe and the Antipodes.

While the BOA members were mainly located in central London and the Home Counties, JM Littlejohn's ability to assist and absorb motley groups from the north and west of England gave his association more balance. Subsequently, the BOA (with never more than 80 US-trained traditionalist members) proceeded to inaugurate their own clinic, which was opened by George Bernard Shaw in 1927.[16] Though numerically small, their influence on their upper class clientele, plus their close AOA connection, gave them immeasurable power within British osteopathic institutions; they were top of an osteopathic pecking order.

Analysis

The events outlined above serve to highlight some of the struggles that beset an alternative medical group who as striving for better courses to equip graduates more effectively and to raise professional standing within communities. Still continued to be seen as the 'Grand Ole Man' ably assisted by his large family who sustained the hopes and prayers of his osteopathic practitioners. His death in 1917 accelerated a reforming cohort to admonish the traditionalist view that the osteopathic lesion was a significant factor in all disease. Yet Still's supporters were harried in the Midwest states by a more dynamic chiropractic profession. JM Littlejohn supported a third way based on a more complicated hypothesis perceiving that much of disease lay in the human condition of adjustment and adaptation. He belived that failure to do so led to disease. Even he was capable of obfuscation in his writings and much of what he intimated was above the comprehension of most of his British colleagues. However, his major practical contribution was to rally small disparate groups of British osteopaths into some cohesion from his position at the helm of his BSO.

References

1.   Hildreth, A.G., *The Lengthening Shadow of Andrew Taylor Still*. Kirksville: Journal Printing. 1938. p.124.
2.   Wharton, J.C., *Nature Cures: the history of alternative medicine in America*. New York: Oxford University Press. 2002. p.141.
3.   Booth, E.R., *History of Osteopathy and Twentieth-Century Medical Practice*. Cincinnati, Ohio: Caxton Press. 1924. pp.92–3.
4.   Ibid., p.546.
5.   Littlejohn College and Hospital, *Prospectus*. 1912–13. p.3.
6.   Kennard, Anne and Sara Littlejohn family interview DVD 2011.
7.   Gevitz, N., Osteopathic Medicine: from deviance to difference. Edited by N. Gevitz, *Other Healers: Unorthodox Medicine in America*. Baltimore: John Hopkins University Press. 1988. pp.142–4.
8.   Gevitz, N., *The DOs*. Baltimore: John Hopkins University Press. 1982. p.90.
9.   Wharton, J.C., p.160.
10.   Gevitz, N., Osteopathic Medicine: from deviance to difference. p.145.
11.   BSO, *Prospectus*. 1924–5. pp.4–5.
12.   BSO, *Prospectus*. 1927–8. p.11. NOA GCRO minutes. p.78.
13.   Kennard, Anne and Sara Littlejohn family interview DVD 2011.
14.   IAO Council meetings 1925–1942 Vol. I. pp.17–19, 21.
15.   Ibid. p.25.
16.   Pheils, M.T., Thank you Mr Shaw. *British Medical Journal*. 1994, 309(6920): 1724–6.

Chapter 4

The First Steps on the Road to State Regulation of British Osteopaths

Précis

Through his lay organisation the Osteopathic Defence League (ODL), the American trained Wilfrid Streeter pressed for state regulation of osteopaths in the UK. American–trained osteopaths under the British Osteopathic Association (BOA) cooperated when their self-interest coincided with Streeter's aims. Meanwhile, JM Littlejohn with his British School of Osteopathy (BSO) and its British-trained graduate association, the Incorporated Association of Osteopaths (IAO), was feeling particularly left out of the events.[1] To complicate matters further, the BOA representatives acted in an arrogant, Machiavellian way by using duplicitous tactics against other osteopathic parties involved in legislation.

Behind the scenes the British Medical Association (BMA) had been meeting regularly to plan its opposition to such a bill. Their preparation and legal tactics were of a highly professional order, overseen and orchestrated during the Select Committee proceedings by OA Hampton, the BMA solicitor. In contrast, the osteopathic defence was ill-conceived, ill-thought out, disunited and fundamentally amateurish. JM Littlejohn's past misdemeanours and the British School of Osteopathy's inadequacies were to be exposed by the opposing counsel. JM Littlejohn was metaphorically crucified and it took another 60 years before this damning episode was redressed

Historical Examination

The American-trained Wilfrid Streeter had a very successful West End practice full of important people and he used his powerful connections to further the cause of state regulation of osteopathy. With Streeter's help and tacit agreement from all interested bodies, WM Adamson MP introduced a Bill in the Commons on 11th February 1931 suggesting that a new osteopathic board should be formed to regulate the practice of osteopathy and to accredit osteopaths. While the Bill was proceeding through the initial stages, the BOA tried to renegotiate its own terms. It demanded majority representation on the board and an amendment to the Bill to give osteopaths the power to issue birth and death certificates, which was an exclusive right for medical practitioners[2] and one that provided both financial rewards and political power. Streeter refused to countenance these amendments, besides which the American-trained osteopaths already had a majority on the board.[3] The BOA declined to support the legislation, stating their belief that the Bill did not stand a hope of being passed. This enmity reached farcical proportions when the BOA proceeded to petition exclusively for a Royal Charter giving its members sole right to use the title 'osteopath' and allowing them to also use the title RO (Registered Osteopath).

An ally, Arthur Greenwood MP, spoke to Lord Palmer, President of the Privy Council, who told him that much opposition to the Bill existed. Greenwood suggested that the BOA meet with the 'medical committee' of the Privy Council to assuage concerns. The BOA subsequently assured the Privy Council that they wanted the Charter, not to increase their medical rights but merely to prevent any unqualified person from using the title 'osteopath'. The Privy Council refused their application citing six counter-petitioners including all three osteopathic co-sponsors of the previous Bill (the ODL, BSO and IAO).[4]

The episode illustrates the utter hopelessness of attempts at united osteopathic legislative enterprise, which was devoid of cohesion, trust, cooperation, mutual respect, good preparation and selflessness. Meanwhile, Sir Herbert Barker, a former osteopathic ally and colleague, was developing a rapprochement among certain medical opponents.

In 1932, James Mennell, an orthopaedic physician at St Thomas's, paid tribute to all manipulators by suggesting that the medical profession could be "warped with prejudice by claims made and dismiss the story told by patients, with a sneer".[5] *The Times* continued this theme by stating that the medical profession could redress past errors by recognising Sir Herbert Barker. Publicly, Streeter pleaded with him not to "make an offer to demonstrate your methods as a *quid pro quo* for recognition". Nonetheless, Barker appeared to distance himself gradually from osteopathy.[6] Streeter felt the loss of Barker's endorsement and friendship. Moreover, osteopathy's opponents effectively exploited this division.[7] It did not help when Barker acknowledged essential differences between bonesetters' methods and osteopathy in a letter to *The Times*.[8]

A further attempt was made to reintroduce the ODL-sponsored Bill in 1933 by Bob Boothby MP but once more it failed to gain momentum. This time all the usual osteopathic supporters gave some lip service to unity.[9] Following the event the American-trained osteopath Dr Mellor stated:

"The BOA could never benefit from contact with the BSO, that equally Osteopathy could not obtain recognition so long as everyone was obliged to go over to the USA to obtain a diploma. It was, therefore, very probable that a Bill would be passed by the medical men to limit osteopaths in their work or to bring manipulation into medicine. It was agreed…to build up the (BOA) clinic."[10]

At least the BOA had now acknowledged the insuperable impasse. The dilemma had been clearly summarised by Neville Chamberlain, Minister of Health in 1926. No British government could agree to state regulation where the majority of affected practitioners worked beyond their jurisdiction. The message was simple and explicit; they needed to establish a British school on the basis of regular medical schools. Further contact did continue with all the parties attending an official dinner in the Commons to inaugurate an Osteopathic Parliamentary Committee. This fragile cooperation resulted in the Bill passing its second reading in the Commons with a proviso that it be referred to a Select Committee of the House of Lords.

While the various osteopathic groups had been patching up their fractious relationship, the medical profession had not been idly sitting back. Medical authorities opposed to the bill to regulate osteopaths consisted of the British Medical Association (BMA) and the Royal Colleges of Physicians and Surgeons involved in strategic planning. It was decided that the BMA would focus on osteopathic credentials, political aspirations and theory, while the Royal Colleges would examine osteopathic scientific data.[11] Meanwhile, the General Medical Council (GMC) would outline a historical perspective of medical professionalisation. The BMA Committee on Osteopathy met for the first time on 4th June 1934.

The BMA's medical secretary George Anderson and his assistant Charles Hill were given responsibility to prepare most of the evidence, while Dr CO Hawthorne was to research osteopathic diagnosis and therapy. Anderson and Hill had started their project six months beforehand. They concluded that British osteopaths wanted a similar status to their American colleagues in the USA. Yet the BMA experts refuted osteopathy's causation of disease theory, which they perceived was based on a narrow biophysical concept of disease that had no scientific basis. Despite many traditional osteopaths ignoring the germ theory and biochemical view of the human process, their disease causation belief had a degree of validity. It was thought by some of the BMA researchers involved in testing osteopathic concepts on spinal conditions that traditionalist theory had some authenticity. Although this osteopathic hypothesis could not be substantiated, an attempted neurophysiological explanation, they considered, was not so foolish.

It was the BMA's view that osteopathic therapy had strength when locally based on certain spinal conditions. However, their curriculum contained most medical subjects and these would by necessity require medical academic staff in order for an approved standard of education to be reached. Realistically, this was untenable for a British osteopathic school. Anderson and Hill's conclusion was that no official recognition was necessary.[12] Hawthorne's report concluded that it was up to osteopaths to establish whether they had discovered an important causative factor of disease.[13] Thus the biophysical concept found expression as the osteopathic lesion. It was seen as osteopaths' responsibility to prove its existence and with the efficacy of manual treatment, to remove it.

American osteopathy was being critically assessed too by the BMA as it had evolved through its pioneering stage (1888–1917), a time when early US osteopathic research, attributed to Louisa Burns and her co-workers, was seriously flawed and lacked any validity.[14] Burns' experiments were contrived to fit osteopathic theory and thus the findings were almost worthless, providing no evidence of the existence of osteopathic lesions or their role as causative factors in disease. Many traditional osteopaths were content to believe in osteopathy without any validation. Yet as American osteopathy entered its post-Still phase (1917–1935), an uneasy debate emerged concerning this distinct lack of valid proof.

A growing number of reforming osteopaths under the leadership of Henry Bunting, editor of the *Osteopathic Physician*, became distinctly critical of this unsubstantiated biophysical concept. One editorial read:

"Would we rather hang on to our dogma that – no matter what the facts show – it has always got to be a mechanical lesion? Nothing is easier to prove in the case of diphtheria, at least, that the word 'mechanical' has no business to be inserted as a necessary condition for getting that disease."[15]

By the late 1930s, osteopathic research under Stedman Denslow reached an acceptable scientific standard.[16] Nevertheless, lack of proof of the lesion and its effects cast doubts in the minds of many osteopaths. This was further exacerbated by limited, anecdotal clinical trials with subjective 'favourable' outcomes. The BMA team was well aware of this dichotomy.

The dilemma that now faced British osteopaths was which direction it should take, either following a more vibrant, evangelical chiropractic profession, pursuing orthodoxy or withering away completely. The American Medical Association gave the BMA valuable information about osteopathy and American osteopathy had been discussed in depth at the BMA Committee on Osteopathy meetings. Information detailing the variable standards of osteopathic education were scrutinised and the controversy between reformers and traditionalists, monitored. They were aware not only of osteopathic competitive struggle with a more tenacious chiropractic profession but also with a more clinically superior medical profession following Flexner's reforms. Moreover, far from being a vibrant osteopathic profession, its predicted decline was imminent.[17] Nevertheless, American osteopathy was benefiting from better collegiate entry standards and a cohort of clinically more discerning practitioners.[18]

At the inception of the BMA Committee on Osteopathy, much discussion concerned implementation of the bill. It was decided that the General Council and Register of Osteopaths (newly founded in 1936) would have policing rights over unregistered practitioners and copyright over specific manipulative techniques. The negatives were that such a system could restrict medical practice and also mean that any cult leader prepared to adopt a standard medical curriculum would have access to state registration.

BMA strategy was to exploit differences between the four osteopathic witnesses. Specific personal profiles of these osteopathic witnesses were drawn up for the legal team to consider.[19] Overall, the BMA team produced high quality research. In comparison, osteopathic preparation was superficial at best, haphazard, naïve, lacking in scholarship, ill-prepared and underfunded.

On 4th March 1935 the Select Committee met for the initial session. Streeter appeared as the first osteopathic witness representing the Osteopathic Defence League (ODL) and took up the first three days. He confirmed to the BMA his "abysmal ignorance…his abysmal ignorance of nature and origin of diseases."[20] Nonetheless, Mrs Chesterton, an ODL supporter present at the hearing, thought that Streeter, "more than held his own but to the lay mind Sir William's (Jowitt) tactics seemed feeble".[21] Part of the third day was taken up with testimony from grateful patients who extolled the fine work carried out by osteopaths. The BMA's solicitor thought Sir William Jowitt, Chief BMA Counsel, performed poorly at this stage[22] and this rather weakened the BMA's position.

The osteopathic witness most feared by the BMA, the eminent Kelman MacDonald, appeared next. The BMA had a dirty dossier on him but decided not to present it.[23] Hempson thought that Jowitt was ineffectual when cross-examining MacDonald on scientific or pseudo-scientific matters, believing that he should have been trying to distance MacDonald from his own osteopathic colleagues, thereby demonstrating the differences between a medical practitioner and his osteopathic counterparts.[24] It was thought that Jowitt should question him on JM Littlejohn, the BSO and the quality of its teaching. He had been briefed that MacDonald, representing American-trained osteopaths, held the BSO in low regard.[25] MacDonald acquiesced to Jowitt's tactics.

Halfway through proceedings on 22th March following MacDonald and three further grateful patients, JM Littlejohn, Dean and proprietor of the British School of Osteopathy was called as a witness.[26] Jowitt had been informed of the poor quality of the BSO, describing it as "a fraudulent establishment ...[whose] standards are despised by the BOA, of which he is a past president." He also asked why JM Littlejohn had left.[27] JM Littlejohn had actually resigned because the BOA had cut all links with his BSO. There is no intimation from surviving archives as to what strategy Jowitt had planned.

On cross-examination Jowitt questioned the validity of Littlejohn's many degrees and doctorates.[28] Littlejohn, described by his osteopathic allies, as a shy, introverted, archetypal absent-minded professor, appeared vacuous, even shifty.[29] Methodically, Jowitt dismantled Littlejohn's PhD, his Doctor of Law and even his MD from Chicago among other academic awards.[30] His family maintain that JM Littlejohn was never really interested in his academic awards or how they were attained and that he was somewhat dumb-founded by this form of interrogation.[31] An eyewitness to the proceedings and avid osteopathic supporter, Mrs Chesterton, stated that it was:

"a deplorable performance ...his failure to recall important facts did not help the case. Indeed, as time went I realised his evidence must have an unfortunate influence on the issue, for the last part of his cross-examination was far worse than the first ...there was a general sense of depression as the interrogation went on."[32]

Jowitt dismantled the academic reputation that Littlejohn had possessed. At the same time the British School of Osteopathy and his altruistic attempts to assist other schools and associations cast severe doubt on its credibility. JM Littlejohn was totally denigrated.[33] The final osteopathic witness representing the Incorporated Association of Osteopaths, Harvey Foote, decided to withdraw.[34] Jowitt had decimated the osteopathic cause for state regulation and the osteopathic legal team rested their case. A whole array of medical experts followed delivering further damning evidence with consummate skill and predictable consequences.[35]

Assuming that the Bill was about to fail, on 5th April 1935 Kelman MacDonald met Viscount Elibank, a supporter, to discuss contingency plans. The rescue strategy was to include: the creation of a voluntary register of osteopaths; the founding of an independent 'trustworthy' school (definitely not the BSO); the pronouncement that all osteopathic students would attend medical schools until the establishment of a full-time course at an osteopathic school with competent educational standards; and those American-trained BOA members who were affiliated to the American Osteopathic Association.[36] When MacDonald was asked whether the Bill could be withdrawn, he informed his BOA colleagues that Elibank was "only putting out feelers" to this effect.

A week later JH Thorpe KC, counsel for osteopathic bodies, read out a statement to the Select Committee stating that the various osteopathic institutions were withdrawing support for the bill. Instead they would be promoting a voluntary register of osteopaths on similar lines to those drawn up by Elibank and MacDonald in that previous meeting. The shell-shocked osteopaths had no notion of either the detailed BMA research undertaken in Britain or the damning scientific and political evidence from America that had been gathered over a year beforehand.

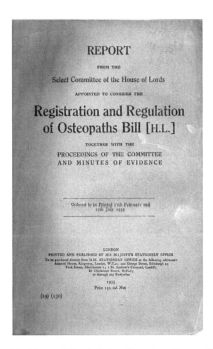

Fig. 13: House of Lords Select Committee Report 1935

Hempson, the BMA solicitor, had been crucial to the events, acting as a puppet-master before, during and after the committee proceedings. He directed events from the sidelines organising the legal team, BMA professional staff and witnesses. Not everything went to plan such as his exasperation of Jowitt's somewhat ineffectual performance during his questioning of grateful patients. Furthermore, Hempson remonstrated with the junior counsel over Jowitt's scientific and pseudo-scientific altercation with MacDonald at the expense of established strategy to isolate MacDonald from his osteopathic colleagues. Nonetheless, it was Jowitt's seemingly spontaneous, devastating coup de grace of Littlejohn's dubious awards in his cross-examination that ultimately lost the osteopaths' support.

The BMA research team had recognised the American osteopathic debate. They exposed osteopathy's narrow, unsubstantiated concept of disease. They were aware that reforming osteopaths were struggling to move scientific osteopathic medicine away from a physical construct based on a lesion, neither the existence of which nor its supposed effects on pathogenesis could be proved. However, the BMA team perceived another crisis in the osteopathic profession; a dilemma of location between chiropractic competition and medical clinical superiority. American medical allies opined the inevitable decline of osteopathy, whose professional and clinical progress had stagnated. It appeared too easy for those witnesses representing the Royal Colleges to refute radiological and osteopathic research based on flawed evidence of the lesion and its pathogenic role. It rather completed a magnificent victory for those against the Bill. Just to drive the message home, two members of the BMA team, Charles Hill and Hugh Clegg, wrote a book for public readership based on their research of osteopathy.[37]

In many ways the debacle reaffirmed the conflict and chasm between each of the rival osteopathic groups. JM Littlejohn protested his innocence and victimisation in the columns of the *Journal of Osteopathy* but he was a broken man. He retired increasingly to Badger Hall and his beloved study where he prepared copious articles in defence of his concepts and of his school. His friends and BSO graduates rallied around making excuses for his suspect degrees, doctorates and dubious BSO diploma[38] but their pronouncements that they had "examined and scrutinised all his diplomas and degrees…[finding them]…beyond adverse criticism" was unconvincing. The House of Lords Select Committee Report stated:

"the only existing establishment in this country for the education and examination of osteopaths was exposed in the course of evidence before us, as being of negligible importance, inefficient for its purpose, and above all, in thoroughly dishonest hands."[39]

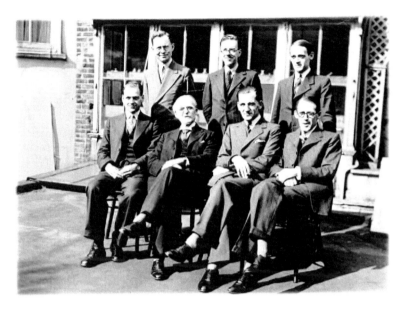

Fig. 14: JM Littlejohn and BSO Faculty

Buoyed by MacDonald's acknowledged performance in the Select Committee report, the BOA felt vindicated.[40] They blamed JM Littlejohn completely for the shambles and maintained a steadfast veto on all matters connected with him and his allied institutions.

Analysis

For all JM's Littlejohn's failings, no British osteopath, least of all BOA members, seemed aware that their failure indicated a paradigm shift in medical education.[41,42] The battle between 'reform' osteopaths and 'traditional' osteopaths would be destined to take place solely in osteopathic teaching hospitals.[43] The progressives decimated their opponents. In a sense, JM Littlejohn's deficiencies had camouflaged the paradigm difference between modern, scientific and 'bedside manner' clinical practice.

Perhaps the best observation was made by one of the progressive's opponents, who suggested opting for a more limited clinical field of activity based on the lines set out by Barker and his bonesetting techniques.[44] He maintained that osteopaths should apply for a modified state regulation similar to dentistry, which was precisely what happened in 1948 at the BSO by Webster-Jones.

JM Littlejohn appeared to be less interested in the day-to-day running of the BSO. He left many of the important decisions to his son, James, an ear, nose and throat surgeon. Another son, Edgar, finished his diploma course at the BSO but never practised, opening instead a bicycle shop in Benfleet, Essex. The youngest, John, did qualify at the BSO and practised into the early 1960s but showed no interest in committee work or teaching.[45] JM Littlejohn's apparent continuing distraction away from the BSO affairs, together with little other family involvement in daily BSO matters, created a hiatus in leadership. This slowly turned into a crisis over the next decade as the issue of who would take over as BSO principal was considered. The BSO progressed through a period of transition, with JM Little-john relinquishing all of his daily responsibilities but remaining titular head of the college until his death in 1947. This period was marked by two distinct influences: a wider interpretation represented by the charismatic but temperamentally de-structive T Edward Hall; and Shilton Webster-Jones (Webber), who together with Clem Middleton and Audrey Smith would reshape the BSO to include JM Littlejohn's biophysical concept reflected in a narrower musculoskeletal apprecia-tion of its worth.

From this post-Littlejohn decade Webber went on to became principal of the BSO, revising the school curriculum to effect these changes. Moreover, scientific inclu-sion led to revised osteopathic subjects and graduates more attune to physical medicine. The debate between pro-BSO and anti-BSO factions would resonate for many decades.

References

1. Littlejohn, J.M., Handwritten notes. BSO archives.
2. Collins, M., *Osteopathy in Britain: the first hundred years*. London: Booksurge. 2005. pp.56–7.
3. Streeter, W.A., *The New Healing*. London: Methuen & Co. 1932. p.230.
4. Ibid., p.232.
5. Streeter, W.A. *The Osteopathic Bulletin*. ODL. No.3. October 1932. p.1. BSO archives.
6. Inglis, B., *Natural Medicine*. London: William Collins & Sons. 1979. p.94.
7. Wells, H.G., Preface. In: Clegg, C. & Hill H.A., *What is Osteopathy?* London: J.M. Dent & Sons Ltd., 1937. p.vii.
8. BMA, 'BMA Legal Notes Drawn up on MacDonald, Littlejohn and Letter in *Times* from Barker.' BMA legal team. 1935.
9. BOA Council minutes 2.5.1933. pp.104–5.
10. Ibid., November 1933. p.116.

11. BMJ, 'What is Osteopathy? And BMA Committee on Osteopathy Appointed.' *British Medical Journal.* Jan–June 3861–3886. 1935. 5.1.1935. p.20.

12. BMA, 'General Osteopathic Political Intentions and Osteopathic Theory.' *BMA Committee on Osteopathy Part 2*, no. Ost. 3. 1934. p.4 & p.9.

13. Hawthorne, C.O., 'Osteopathy as a Diagnostic and Therapeutic Method.' *BMA Committee on Osteopathy Part 3*, no. Ost. 4. 1934. p.3.

14. House of Lords Select Committee, *Registration and Regulation of Osteopaths Bill.* London: H.M. Stationery Office, 1935. p.451 nos. 6253–4.

15. Gevitz, N., *The DOs.* Baltimore: John Hopkins University Press. 1982. pp.90–3.

16. Ibid., pp.90–2.

17. BMA, 'Quality of Osteopathic Education in the USA.' *BMA Committee on Osteopathy Part 4*, no. Ost 16. 1.2.1935. pp.1–3.

18. BMA, 'Quality of Osteopathic Education in the USA.' *BMA Committee on Osteopathy Part 4*, no. Ost 17. 1.2.1935. pp.6–7.

19. BMA, 'BMA Legal Notes Drawn up on MacDonald, Littlejohn.' BMA legal team. 1935.

20. BMA., 'O.A. Hempson: correspondence re Osteopathic Bill (1935)' from OAH to Jowitt. 7.3.1935.

21. Chesterton, C., *This Body: an experience in osteopathy.* London: Stanley Paul & Co, 1937. pp.108–112, 131.

22. BMA, 'O.A. Hempson: correspondence. O.A.H. to Anderson, 23.4.(3?).1935.

23. OAH to 'Hal' Dicken (junior counsel), 23.3.1935.

24. BMA, A letter to O.A. Hempson informing him of the death of one of MacDonald's female patients.

25. BMA. 'O.A. Hempson: correspondence. Charles Hill to OAH. 22.3.1935.

26. Ibid.

27. BMA, 'BMA Legal Notes Drawn up on MacDonald, Littlejohn etc.' p.1.

28. House of Lords Select Committee, *Registration and Regulation of Osteopaths Bill.* pp.221–8.

29. General Council and Register of Osteopaths, *The Osteopathic Blue Book: the origin and development of osteopathy in Great Britain.* London: GCRO. 1957. pp.17–21

30. Flexner, A., *The Flexner Report.* 1910. p.216. 'The city of Chicago in respect to medical education is the plague spot for education.'

31. Kennard Anne & Sara Littlejohn family interview DVD 2011.

32. Chesterton, pp.132–6.

33. General Council and Register of Osteopaths, p.19.

34. IAO Council minutes 13.7.1935. pp. 27–8.

35. BMJ, Leading article 'successful campaign'. *British Medical Journal.* Vol. no.1. Jan–June 3861–3886. 1935. pp.832–3.

36. BOA Council minutes. 5.4.1935. pp.149–50.

37. Clegg, H.A. & Hill, C., *What is Osteopathy?* London: J.M. Dent & Sons Ltd. 1937.

38. Collins, pp.144–5.

39. General Council and Register of Osteopaths, p.19.
40. House of Lords Select Committee, p.v. clause 7.
41. Gevitz, N., Osteopathic Medicine: from deviance to difference. Edited by N. Gevitz, *Other Healers: Unorthodox Medicine in America*. Baltimore: John Hopkins University Press. 1988. pp.138–9.
42. Ibid.
43. Gevitz, N., *The DOs*. pp.93–4.
44. Graham-Little MP, E., *British Medical Journal*, Vol. no.1. Jan-Jun 3861–3886. 1935. pp.96–7.
45. Kennard, Anne and Sara family interview DVD 2011.

Chapter 5

The General Council and Register of Osteopaths in the Early Years: Success or Failure?

Précis

The General Council and Register of Osteopaths (GCRO) was primarily established as a voluntary register for all fully qualified osteopaths. Unfortunately, some British Osteopathic Association (BOA) members viewed its foundation as a hegemonic prize for MacDonald's splendid performance in the Select Committee proceedings. A third of the BOA membership perceived the GCRO as an irrelevance and refused to join the Register, after all, the BOA already gave them supposedly superior registration rights. Be that as it may, three American-trained osteopathic officials of this newly formed voluntary GCRO guided their British-trained colleagues towards majority membership, and significantly, to majority control of the Register, much to the chagrin of their American-trained counterparts. The Incorporated Association of Osteopaths (IAO), recently renamed the Osteopathic Association of Great Britain (OAGB) and its GCRO-accredited BSO, not only became the majority on the Register, but its representation on the GCRO council outstripped their BOA colleagues.

Within a decade, many BOA members had resigned or been expelled for failing to pay GCRO membership fees. Their own postgraduate school, The London College of Osteopathy (founded in 1946), and its alumni drifted towards the British Association of Manipulative Medicine (BAMM) and an unsuccessful tie up with the British Medical Association via the Osteopathic Medical Association (OMA). Meanwhile, the British Naturopathic Association (BNA) with its recently founded British College of Naturopathy (BCN), sought some kind of rapprochement with the GCRO, whilst the Register continued to sue, over a protracted period, a BNA member for self-styling himself as a "Registered Osteopath". The High Court award against the BNA member scuppered any chance of conviviality between the parties.

The BNA changed its name to the British Naturopathic and Osteopathic Association (BNOA) and the school to the British College of Naturopathy and Osteopathy (BCNO) founded in 1947. Its members and alumni were able to designate themselves "Registered

Naturopath and Osteopath", much to the irritation of the GCRO council, which had expended a great deal of time and finances on the High Court ruling. Although skirmishes perpetuated for some decades, there was a mutual realisation that further High Court action could bankrupt both the BNOA and GCRO and certain dialogue did take place in the late 1970s and early 1980s.

Historical Examination

The GRCO was set up in 1936 by a number of individuals including Viscount Elibank (who was pro-osteopathy and on the Select Committee), Kelman Mac-Donald, Wilfrid Streeter and the US-trained osteopath Harvey Foote. MacDonald, registrar of the voluntary GCRO, believed that the Register should be run by a council of five members who would "govern all their future activities and determine their status". The IAO had been renamed the Osteopathic Association of Great Britain (OAGB) and it was hoped that their members would individually apply for membership. It was queried whether OAGB members should be given full or associate status with no voting rights.[1] Even though their support was crucial to the Register's success, OAGB members were not afforded the same privileges as those of the BOA, who were automatically accepted en bloc without having to undergo individual scrutiny. It was deemed that BOA members could be appointed as part of the five member governing committee, something which was denied to others.[2]

Harvey Foote advised against an OAGB boycott of the Register.[3] His opinion to fellow OAGB members was that MacDonald and Streeter would find it inconceivable to officiate over a Register of Osteopaths consisting primarily of two thirds of BOA members only. Moreover, Foote sensed that if individual GCRO applications were made by OAGB officials with the hope of gaining full membership in due course, eventually it would lead to en bloc OAGB registration and finally, GCRO accreditation of the BSO.

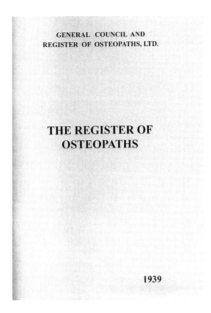

GENERAL COUNCIL AND
REGISTER OF OSTEOPATHS, LTD.

THE REGISTER OF OSTEOPATHS

1939

Fig. 15: GCRO Directory 1939

The table below details information on membership of the first Register of Osteopaths in 1939. By then there were 139 full members and 17 Associates.[4] The domination of British-trained osteopaths over their American counterparts is clear to see.

Date of Entry	US-trained	UK-trained	NSO	Independents
12.3.1937	14	*	*	*
	19	3 (OAGB)	*	*
1.4.1938	11	41 (OAGB)	6	3
	*	1 (BSO)	8 Associates	*
(?1).12.1938	1	29 (OAGB)	5 Associates	4 Associates
	*	11 (BSO)	*	*
Total	**45**	**85**	**6 plus 13 Associates**	**3 plus 4 Associates**

Table 5.1: Members on the first Register of Osteopaths, 1939
(* = data not available)

Harvey Foote's words were heeded. The OAGB leadership convinced a large number of its membership to apply for a place on the Register against much sustained and vitriolic opposition from others, led by T Edward Hall, vice-dean of the BSO. Two tranches of OAGB/BSO applicants were successful in obtaining full membership and this group remained dominant on the GCRO until the early 1980s. However, MacDonald does deserve some credit in opposing his BOA colleagues, for resisting change and preventing Viscount Elibank, the GCRO president, from resigning. In time, Foote (before his early death), MacDonald and Streeter steered the direction of the Register away from being a failed institution to one with the potential for development.

It was hoped that individual applications from members of the National Society of Osteopaths (comprising of 60–100 people largely from the non-accredited New Jersey School of Osteopathy, New York, and some independent practitioners) would give the GCRO a more diverse base. In fact, few reached the standard necessary to join. Without GCRO officials' intervention the Register would have ended up in a BOA backwater as a postscript to osteopathic enmity.[5] Accreditation of the BSO provided some opportunity too. After all, it had been vilified in the Select Committee Report together with JM Littlejohn's tenure as dean.

It is slightly mystifying that JM Littlejohn handed over his 80% of shares in the BSO to an independent board of trustees,[6] something he had obstinately refused to even contemplate twelve years earlier. His family seem to think that JM Littlejohn was kindly disposed towards the GCRO officials involved in talks about transferring BSO control to independent trustees.[7] However, it has to be said that the Littlejohn brothers probably made a good profit from their Chicago College from course fees, treatments carried out at the school's clinics and the sale of the college. JM Littlejohn's purchase of the Badger Hall estate, Thundersley, Essex and his central London flat (leased in 1913) had required a considerable amount of money. One must take into account too that even by 1926, the BSO's potential revenue was yet to be realised. Twelve years later, much of the Littlejohn private family money had been used to finance BSO student loans, a vast amount of which was never repaid.[8] After the House of Lords Select Committee Report, JM Littlejohn retreated to his study and none of his children had any intention of taking on his burdensome mantle.

Disharmony continued into the Second World War. The BOA remained suspicious of OAGB/BSO intent during 1940, and a further skirmish occurred over the province of Ontario's recognition of the BSO as a bona fide osteopathic college. Five years earlier, the BOA had succeeded in persuading the province to temporarily delete the BSO from its list of approved osteopathic colleges. Now the BSO complained to the GCRO over the more recent BOA's reactivation of a ban on the school.

Jocelyn Proby in Canada wrote to his BOA colleagues beseeching them not to further damage the reputation of an accredited GCRO school, especially when one of the parties responsible for GCRO membership was undermining the only British recognised school. The BOA replied to the GCRO that it may have indeed recognised and accredited the BSO but the BOA certainly had not. It showed that some BOA members had little faith in cooperating with their BSO colleagues on the GCRO and by 1950 many of them had resigned or refused to pay their GCRO fees in arrears.

The attempts to restore a unified front dissipated in rancour. BOA members such as Jocelyn Proby, Sammy Ball and Philip Jackson did become GCRO chairmen, but they were the exceptions rather than the rule. Meanwhile, American osteopathic medicine emerged from six Flexner-reforming schools and their upgraded teaching hospitals. From that time onwards, no American-trained graduates considered emigrating to Britain in order to establish narrower manipulative practises there. American-trained traditionalists opened their own postgraduate college in London in 1946 but few medical graduates took up the opportunity and those that did were not entirely enthused to join the GCRO. Moreover, these medical osteopaths saw their future ties as lying with the British Association of Manipulative Medicine (BAMM) and their newly formed Osteopathic Medical Association (OMA), which tried unsuccessfully to associate with the British Medical Association (BMA).

The creation of the National Health Service had a huge impact on British osteopathy. In one step, private patient choice was removed. Under the NHS, treatment was free at the point of access. No longer could professionals treat NHS patients unless they were registered medical practitioners or were under their supervision.[9]

By the 1950s, the number of BOA US-trained osteopaths and postgraduate trained medics at the London College of Osteopathy on the GCRO had dwindled. In contrast, the GCRO went out of its way to ensure some degree of partiality by offering the BOA head, Dora Sutcliffe Lean, ex-officio representation on its council. The proposal was refused dramatically. Dr Lean resigned from the GCRO with some of her BOA colleagues, resurrecting earlier animosity towards the BSO-dominated institution. Ironically, her pretext had been over GCRO legal activities preventing unregistered osteopaths using the title "Registered Osteopath". Such a position appeared inconsistent with her previous views. Alongside, the BOA made no attempt to inform LCO alumni of GCRO presence.[10] Indeed, the GCRO showed signs of considerable professional capability fortified by its long-serving Registrar, Richard Miller, who had joined the Register under GCRO clause 11 (this provision which closed in 1951 allowed practitioners to undergo testing to assess their proficiency for entry to the GCRO). Ironically, Miller and Sir William Elliot, its new president, provided new standards of proficiency at council meetings: to effectively free the log-jam of recurring matters and talent spot younger colleagues for promotion to the council, namely people like Colin Dove and Donald Norfolk.

During the 1960s, Miller and Elliot addressed the role of the GCRO and how its activity overlapped with other institutions. It appeared that all associated organisations "have 142 committee appointments to be filled out of the total of 247 members". Practically, only a few colleagues gave sufficient time to sit on these committees; diverse professional bodies were represented by a small quorum of members. Consequently, the GCRO suggested to various groups that pooling administrative resources would liberate many of the duplicated roles and result in less squandering of effort, alleviate pressure, but would also enable them to continue to uphold their independent status. However, the GCRO was prepared to go it alone. If other groups disagreed with this notion they could provide a secretariat for their own purposes by raising membership subscriptions. However, one institution, the BSO, was prepared to share some staff.[11]

In 1962 an administrative officer, Commander Michael Morris RN (Retd),[12] was appointed on a salary of £1250.00 (which increased by £100.00 one month later). There is a custom in this country to provide ex-service officers with employment on 'Civvy Street'. It is deemed that they bring attributes such as chain of command experience, the ability to speak publicly, loyalty, degrees of integrity and confidence to an organisation. Be that as it may, it is a matter of debate whether these characteristics can actually be successfully applied to the wider world of commerce and the professions.

Anecdotally, Michael Morris exemplified this enigma. His office was located in the subterranean bowels of the BSO, 16 Buckingham Gate, London, SW1. On one wall, a large map of Britain projected similar coloured flags, pinpointing specific GCRO members geographically. Another set of flags indicated the location of our naturopathic colleagues, akin to those used in the Battle of Britain during the Second World War. A florid, somewhat irascible character, Morris brought his own version of naval eccentricity to the proceedings. Viewing our naturopathic fraternity and sorority as the enemy, he rather fuelled animosity between different groups. Periodically, he would take leave to participate in Royal Naval Reserve activities and inevitably his paranoia was increased, casting serious doubts within the GCRO.

Morris' inflexible disposition overshadowed the mid-1960s review of the GCRO and OAGB and their overlapping activities. It was proposed by the GCRO to amalgamate with the OAGB so as to prevent as much duplication as possible. Morris was delegated to put the GCRO case to the OAGB president. Donald Norfolk and Gordon Beech who had duel council representation, were instructed to seek the opinion of their OAGB colleagues. "It was pointed out that the matter, relative to GCRO-OAGB was a delicate one, requiring considerable diplomacy to bring an amalgamation into being."[13] Much discussion took place, but Donald Norfolk held the view that his association had the task of defending its members whereas the primary function of the Register was protecting the public. He suggested that it was a question of demarcating these dissimilar roles rather than fusing the two bodies together. Furthermore, he expressed the view that members regarded the GCRO as "a rather strict body whereas the association was a friendly one".[14]

Morris' attempt at steamrollering the amalgamation through without heeding Norfolk's concerns culminated in a farcical situation on 11th November 1966. That Friday morning, the OAGB AGM voted by 56 votes to 46 for an amendment against amalgamation.[15] In the afternoon at the same Eccleston Hotel during a session of the GCRO AGM, a motion to amalgamate both bodies was carried, even though 95% of the GCRO had this duel membership and some of those who voted against amalgamation in the morning changed their mind in the afternoon! The membership had been confused first by Norfolk's oratory in the morning and then by Morris' behind-the-scenes conspiratorial attempts to persuade GCRO voters otherwise. Not insisting on the GCRO AGM taking place *prior* to the OAGB AGM in order to carry a successful pro-amalgamation consensus forward to the OAGB assembly was a great error. Norfolk and his supporters must have realised that the morning anti-amalgamation vote was incisive. It didn't matter if the vote went in favour of an amalgamation recommendation at the GCRO's afternoon meeting as the OAGB vote against precluded any decision taken in the afternoon anyway.

Morris, some of his GCRO council colleagues and a significant number of members, reacted badly to this situation. Animosity between officials of both bodies increased resentment and a number resigned from the OAGB. Later on, a growing disparity between the two bodies, also involving competition for members' insurance-to-practice services, created further rancour. GCRO professionalism continued to grow, if somewhat haphazardly, and Morris deserves some credit for this. However, his efforts could have been more effective if he had couched them with more flexible diplomacy. Moreover, Richard Miller, a longstanding Registrar and successful GCRO clause 11 applicant, should have been more concerned with reopening clause 11 for others, especially naturopathic osteopaths.

In the early 1950s, a certain William H Dodd of Stourbridge, Worcestershire applied to join the GCRO but was rejected.[16] Undeterred, he advertised as a Registered Naturopath and Registered Osteopath. In response, the GCRO took legal action to prevent him from doing so, which resulted in High Court proceedings. Delays took place, partly due to Dodd's counsel trying to obtain 'security of costs' against the GCRO and also caused by the Register's fear of raising sufficient funds to mount such action.[17] The GCRO had explained to Dodd's legal advisors that they had no qualms about him calling himself an osteopath but "Registered Osteopath" was not acceptable as it conferred membership of the GCRO. It was this point of law up for verification by the High Court. The GCRO council also corresponded with and met face-to-face British Naturopathic Association (BNA) council members. These proceedings took place in a positive atmosphere, it was agreed that "the door was open" for future discussions and a more formally structured meeting took place one year on.[18]

Meanwhile, Dodd's case trundled on. It was proceeding towards an outcome and the legal costs for a one day action were estimated at 2,250 guineas. As the end came into sight there was a distinct lack of reciprocal communication from the BNA. Moreover, GCRO membership was also troubled by the duration of the lawsuit and this was not helped by news of Dodd's serious illness, which created a degree of urgency and despondency. By early 1960, the BNA was prepared to meet up with the GCRO, even though the lawsuit against their member was to proceed in that year. A joint meeting took place and it was agreed that Sir William Elliot would chair subsequent gatherings and future agenda would be drawn up on a more formal, business-like level.[19]

Eventually, after an incredible six years of preparation, the High Court proceedings were all over in a matter of an hour or two. Dodd's defence team withdrew and acceded to Dodd not calling himself "Registered Osteopath". The whole process had cost an immense amount of money and time to prepare. What appeared to have been a magnificent gain for GCRO members turned out to be a pyrrhic victory.[20] By the autumn, the BNA had severed all connections with the GCRO, adjourning all future meetings. Yet both the names of the BNA and the British College of Naturopathy were changed by the addition of the word Osteopath(y). They informed all members that they were entitled to use "Registered Naturopath and Osteopath" and the GCRO was powerless to do a thing about it.

The ludicrous episode wasted money and effort which either side could ill-afford, also serving to perpetuate various myths within the profession that continued for a further three decades. Indeed, meetings took place but there came gradual mutual realisation that the term "Registered Osteopath" could not be defended and at least four members of the BNOA used that title openly. The GCRO appealed to the BNOA council to admonish their members for doing so. The truth was that both parties were fully aware that another High Court action on similar grounds could well bankrupt them both. The implications brought both of them to their senses and some sort of neutral position (neither hostile nor amicable) was reached. By the 1970s and 1980s levels of intolerance were disappearing and the GCRO had become ready to explore dialogue, but trust and cooperation were still not in evidence.

Analysis

The idea of a voluntary register, the GCRO, emerged from talks between Kelman MacDonald and Lord Elibank during sittings of the Select Committee of the House of Lords. Both realised that any chance of statutory regulation was inconceivable after Sir William Jowitt, BMA Counsel, had destroyed its chances, following his metaphorical destruction of JM Littlejohn and his BSO. It was among this debris that the GCRO came into being with three American-trained osteopaths at its helm under the presidency of Viscount Elibank. Initial recruitment took in any member of the BOA en bloc. However, only two thirds joined and many of these only half-heartedly. They perceived that their own association provided the majority of tasks, which were simply just duplicated by the Register. Moreover, other osteopathic groups were not allowed the same favour and they could apply as individuals only. These groups included: graduates of the BSO, not members of the OAGB; OAGB members; National Society of Osteopaths, mainly graduates of non-accredited American Osteopathic Association colleges; and independent nona-ligned osteopaths. All in all it was not a good start from an organisation supposed to treat all osteopaths fairly in a non-discriminatory way.

Due to practical considerations and some altruism, MacDonald, Streeter and Foote constructed a strategy to accept non-aligned BSO graduates and OAGB members in two tranches to become registered with full voting rights. In three years, following the Register's inception, BSO graduates and its alumnae association became its majority of members. Consequently, discouraged registered BOA members started to resign or were dismissed for not paying their outstanding prescriptions but more importantly, their own number were diminishing, caused by the fact that no American-trained osteopaths emigrated to Britain after the Second World War. The Register became for all intents and purposes, a BSO institution, tainted further by the GCRO locating to the BSO basement and sharing office staff. Ironically, its longstanding Registrar, Richard Miller, had joined under GCRO memorandum clause 11, which allowed non-accredited school graduates to apply for membership via an examination. This clause was abolished in the early

1950s. Miller appeared to stand in the way of any entente cordiale with other groups. Thus, from its origin, Miller maintained its ethos of continuing discrimination and predication among its osteopathic community.

GCRO presence, like the curate's egg, has been good in parts. It had been too partisan, too divisive, obstructive and inward looking. However, at the same time it had also brought a group of individuals practising a rural trade towards greater professionalism and played a part in the evolution of osteopathy.

1. Collins, M., *Osteopathy in Britain: the first hundred years.* London: Booksurge. 2005. pp.150–7.
2. GCRO Council minutes 12.3.1937. pp.77–8. The applications came under four headings, BOA (automatic approval and only group who could become council members); OAGB; National Society of Osteopaths (NSO); and Independents, individual persons.
3. OAGB Council minutes 3.10.1936.
4. General Osteopathic Council archives: *Analysis of 1939 Register of Members and Associate Members* carried out in 1953. It contains 21 associates, but only 17 can be countered. Associates were allowed to practise, but had no voting rights. Full members: 85 OAGB/BSO members can be established from records. There were three initially: Milne, van Straten and Saul; GCRO Council minutes 1.4.38 pp.118–120, 41 OAGB and 1, Dr Carloss did not possess a BSO diploma because he had not paid all his school fees. BOA members 45 (cannot make 51 as in the 1953 *Analysis*). National Society of Osteopaths, 6 and individual members unaffiliated to any association, 3.
5. NOA GCRO/CO/Minutes/File 1 pp.78–80.
6. Ibid., p.149.
7. Kennard, Anne and Sara Littlejohn family interview DVD 2011.
8. Ibid.
9. South Wales Osteopathic Society, *History of Osteopathy in Britian.* http://www.osteopathywales.com/index.php?option=com_content&view=article&id=143:history-of-osteopathy-in-britain&catid=15:osteopathy-articles-.
10. NOA GCRO/CO/Minutes file 2. 8 March 1958. p.2.
11. Ibid. 21 April 1961. p.2.
12. Ibid. 24 February 1962. p.1.
13. Ibid. 9 July 1965. pp.2–3.
14. Ibid. 2 March 1966. Pp.2–3.
15. NOA OAGB/Council/AGM/FILE 1. 11 Nov 1966. pp.5–18.
16. NOA GCRO/CO/Minutes/File 1 p.492.
17. NOA GCRO/CO/Minutes/File 2. 23 February 1957 pp.2–3.

18. Ibid., 8 March 1958 pp.1–2; 10 December 1958 p.4; 7 February 1959; 21 March 1959 p.1; 25 July 1959. p.3; 21 November 1959 pp.1–3; 20 February 1960 p.1; 9 July 1960 pp.1–2.

19. NOA/GCRO/CO/Minutes 8 March 1958 pp.1–2.

20. Ibid. AGM 21 April 1961. pp.2–4.

Chapter 6

The British School of Osteopathy in the Middle of the Twentieth Century

Précis

From 1935, JM Littlejohn, once cast as a reluctant guru of British-trained osteopaths, started to very slowly but surely disengage from day-to-day events at the British School of Osteopathy (BSO) although his lecturing workload continued. He instigated James, his ENT surgeon son, to negotiate matters of importance. JM Littlejohn was after all 70 years of age and entitled to slow down, but unfortunately his reputation outside the organisation and the Osteopathic Association of Great Britain (OAGB) had become somewhat tarnished after the House of Lords Select Committee Report. He began to retreat, evermore increasingly, to his study at Badger Hall, to write articles in defence of his name. Neither of his younger sons – Edgar nor John, both BSO graduates – showed any inclination to take on the onerous tasks of financing and running the BSO.

The resultant hiatus of leadership at the BSO had implications that reverberated for the next 13 years on the appointment of Shilton Webster-Jones (Webber), and continued to cause ructions for a further 17 years and even beyond. Moreover, the obstructive shadow of T Edward Hall, vice-dean and emerging guru, hung heavily over its destiny during much of the next three decades. In the 1950s, Webster-Jones, Clem Middleton, Audrey Smith together with Margot Gore and Colin Dove pooled their talents to provide the BSO with enough cohesion to sustain its precarious position in spite of all short-comings.[1] Their efforts delivered a blueprint for other colleges to adopt beyond the next century.

Historical Examination

Before the findings of the House of Lords Select Committee meetings were published, T Edward Hall wrote a piece for *Time & Tide* magazine about the proceedings. His letter berated British Osteopathic Association (BOA) representatives and Kelman MacDonald in particular for disabusing the BSO, whilst at the same time he hurled some more brickbats at American-trained colleagues.[2] His emerging presence as BSO vice-dean and OAGB council member was extremely forthright, to say the least. His manner was especially noticeable during sensitive talks when negotiating an en bloc entry pathway for members and BSO accreditation and between the OAGB and the newly established voluntary General Council and Register of Osteopaths (GCRO).

Hall was the Dr Jekyll and Mr Hyde of Osteopathy. On the one hand he was a person of charisma, charm and generosity, but his dark side possessed an erratic, disruptive nature. Hall's legacy was to achieve acclamation and defamation in equal amounts. His emotional fluctuations appear to have been fuelled by alcohol and hereditary factors. From family correspondence we are aware that his sister, Florence Hall, suffered from periods of chronic depression and anxiety leading to dementia. Edward himself might well have suffered from a less prominent but similar psychosis, probably exacerbated by alcohol.[3] Nevertheless, he was a brilliant technician, complimenting a thorough knowledge of musculoskeletal anatomy with a successful West End London practice. Before training as an osteopath, Hall had been a successful professional musician in a band. During that time he must have been aware of the essential role of solo instrumentalists, as both swaying band members but also more importantly, its audience.

The gifted Hall was no academic and exposure to JM Littlejohn's more academic qualities only served to strengthen Hall's clinical technical expertise. Four decades before, protestations to AT Still led to the injection of more medical subjects into a limited Kirksville curriculum, at the expense of osteopathic matters. The apparently ironic plea for more medical subjects to be studied at the sacrifice of osteopathic ones would reverberate incessantly down the ages, even though JM Littlejohn and his fellow Scots were defeated for suggesting modifications to the course which did not preclude greater osteopathic intervention.[4] Still was well aware that his osteopathic leadership had been threatened. His response was to utter this conceivable, inscrutable expression: osteopathy is not apart from nature but a part of nature. Hall was, in essence, a true descendent of good-time Still osteopathy who offered practical, confident, lightning bonesetting. The problem with this familiar call for "more osteopathy/less medicine" does not appear to have had much coherence in reality.

Did osteopathy require a belief system central to its ethos? Some considered this to be the case. It is a perfectly reasonable view if one is prepared to see osteopathy as a religion guided by a god. It was also possible to believe in osteopathy in a purely secular sense based on supposition. Despite being a former minister JM Littlejohn was a believer in osteopathy and the path of rational explanation he followed was a more difficult, tortuous journey.

If alive today, would JM Littlejohn have been content to see that no one had ventured outside his route? It is unlikely he would have guessed that the only

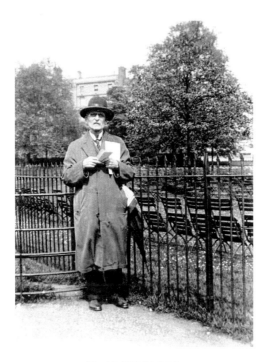

Fig. 16: JM Littlejohn

progression osteopathy would take was the adoption of new techniques. The profession has never had a tradition of challenging different hypotheses in an atmosphere of academic thoroughness and in the absence of personal acrimony. A lack of open-minded testing of principles, premises and suppositions can lead to a diminution and, perhaps, the stagnation of scholarship, perception and even integrity. The role of a guru who upholds a belief system, a set of principles, conjecture and techniques, has a special place for many but it should not displace reasoned analysis or review.

Traditionally, osteopathy had been guided by gurus, starting with the charismatic and driven AT Still. Even the academic JM Littlejohn became a reluctant guru to those rallying around the BSO in those early days. Eventually, T Edward Hall fulfilled many of the attributes required. He possessed great physical presence, was an adept technician, a formidable performer and his resonant Lancastrian voice emphasised these skills. Here was a guru of a different form but a leader nonetheless, rallying the membership following the Select Committee debacle. Hall appeared to take up the challenge for BSO-trained osteopaths at the very time when JM Littlejohn was faltering.

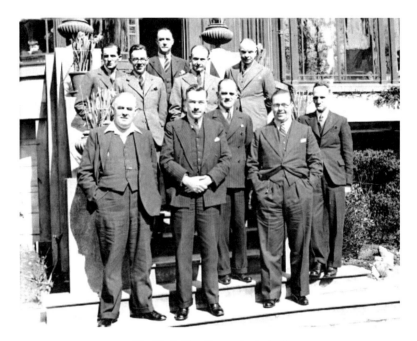

Fig. 17: OAGB Convention in 1937

In 1938, Hall was BSO vice-dean, president of the OAGB, and, seemingly, JM Littlejohn's heir-apparent but this was not endorsed as far as the Littlejohn family was concerned.[5] His wife, the medical graduate Dr Dorothy Wood, gave support to him and also to the BSO. According to records he was unafraid to vent his feelings, citing a series of "small incidents over a long period of time". Some tried to dissuade him from resignation but he was adamant.[6] Thus began a recurring theme of his tenure at the BSO. Meanwhile, JM Littlejohn's health deteriorated to such an extent that he was no longer capable of fulfilling his BSO lectureship responsibilities anymore and these activities were taken over by Clem Middleton and Shilton Webster-Jones (Webber). The duo ran the BSO diligently through the worst period of the Second World War. By 1943, the American-trained Jocelyn Proby had been contacted by a frail JM Littlejohn to act as deputy Dean of the BSO and its Board of governing directors, following Hall's resignation from the BSO Board. When Proby found life too difficult in war-torn London, Hall was appointed in his place as vice-dean and member of the BSO board, without any appreciation of Hall's vitriolic reputation.

The decision created consternation among some of the BSO faculty and subsequently, Middleton and Webber resigned from the BSO as Director of Clinic duties and Registrar respectively. Neither of them felt they could work with Hall. At this time, Webber had been legally advised not to express his personal views that Hall was an alcoholic schizophrenic.[7] We can only surmise that his marriage to Dorothy Wood was deteriorating badly (it would eventually end in divorce), irrevocably contributing to his fragile mental state.[8] Equally, we can only postulate JM Littlejohn's intervention on the matter of Hall's installation. JM Littlejohn's letters to Middleton and Webber beseeching them to reconsider their positions might well have been more decisive if his health had been more robust. Nevertheless, both were elevated to the BSO's board, which gave them considerable influence to nullify Hall's interventions. Later, Webber was appointed vice-dean in 1947 after another Hall resignation.[9] Hall could be obstructive, haphazard, ultrasensitive and, on occasions, somewhat paranoid.

The whole affair not only acted as a precursor for succession at the BSO but also marked a change in the direction of British osteopathy. This struggle, unknowingly, was an internecine scrap, a guru versus consensus-led group. Inherent in new movements, gurus play an important part in gathering supporters to maintain momentum while the 'crusade' develops. In time, some of these new supporters unconsciously threaten this order by rivalling the leader, in time becoming mini-gurus themselves. Displaying technical/clinical prowess was the usual way for osteopaths to demonstrate their authority. College technique and clinical departments existed as separate entities within a school, rather endorsing this activity. The technique faculty acted autonomously while the clinic faculty never effectively acted synchronously with the academic side. Promotion to senior collegiate positions was well within grasp for those technically astute and ambitious enough to desire it. Indeed, a technique and clinic faculty could foster in its tutors a sense of accomplished manipulative finesse couched in esoteric mystery and awe without any application to specific disorders. 'We treat people, not conditions' was one of the brief ripostes used to put new recruits or students firmly in their places.

Hall was able to maintain a toehold teaching technique at the BSO, whilst at the same time openly criticising to students its management, direction and ethos. In contrast, Webber showed that the institution required the collective cohesion, stamina, durability and tolerance offered by a small group of people committed to the BSO. Gurus alone cannot provide these factors on a regular basis whilst repeatedly asking to resign if matters presuppose. Yet, in osteopathic hagiography, the guru will be remembered over successful administrators, academics and principals.

Webber was appointed BSO principal on JM Littlejohn's death in 1948. This event heralded a turning point in the annals of UK osteopathy. Webber, Middleton and Audrey Smith along with Margot Gore and Colin Dove began to change the BSO in an orderly, constructive way. The group reorganised the curriculum to include only those conditions which seemed to benefit from osteopathy. In the main these were musculoskeletal conditions along the lines surprisingly advocated by Sir Herbert Barker and E Graham-Little MP.[10] Nevertheless, Hall's brooding presence was always around to oppose these innovations as part of an anti-BSO faction. Hall finally severed his ties with the school in 1964 but managed to emerge as a figurehead of traditional osteopathy with Continental European roots. Webber would later reflect that it was never his intention to jettison JM Littlejohn's contributions, but rather to set aside those contentious matters until osteopathy had been more accepted by the general public.

The table below outlines variation in the curricula studied over time. It is in the 3rd and 4th years that the greatest changes are visible.

	1936–7[11]	Early 1950s[12]
2nd Year	Anatomy	Anatomy (and embryology)
	Physiology	Physiology (and histology)
	Bacteriology	Applied Anatomy (part 1 somatic)
	Introduction – Osteopathy & Clinical Diagnosis	Introduction to Osteopathy
	Introduction to Principles	
	Introduction to Osteopathic Movement	
3rd Year	Osteopathic Principles & Diagnosis	Osteopathic Principles & Diagnosis
	Osteopathic Practice	Osteopathic Practice (3rd & 4th years)
	Osteopathic Technique	Osteopathic Technique
	Dietetics	Dietetics
	Osteopathic Applied Anatomy	Applied Anatomy of the Foot
	Spinal Physiological Movements	Pathology (3rd & 4th years)
	Pharmacology	Neurology
	Medical & Surgical Diagnosis	Orthopaedics
4th Year	Applied Anatomy & Physiology	Applied Anatomy (part 2)
	Osteopathic Technique	Osteopathic Technique
	Osteopathic Practice	Osteopathic Practice
	Minor Surgery	Minor Surgery
	Psychotherapeutics	Psychology

	ENT	ENT
	Pediatrics (sic)	Paediatrics
	Gynaecology & Obstetrics	Gynaecology
	Osteopathic Specialities	Specialities
		Pathology
		Comparative Therapeutics
		Medical (clinical) Diagnosis
		Surgical Diagnosis
		The Eye in General Practice
		Skin

Table 6.1: Comparison of Subjects Studied at the BSO in 1936/7 and the Early 1950s

Later, Webber appointed postgraduate medical staff who were preparing for their Membership and Fellowship consultancy exam to instruct basic medical subjects at a high level, giving BSO students a thorough grounding in essential medical sciences.[13] Webber's reforms set the seal for cohorts of osteopaths to enter practice with a more comprehensive appreciation of biophysical medicine.

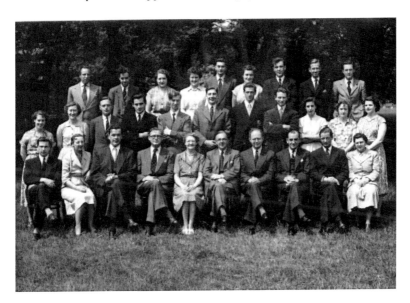

Fig. 18: BSO in 1957

In 1968, Colin Dove took over as BSO principal with Audrey Smith supplementing an extra year to the curriculum. It was Dove who promoted a more varied biopsychosocial concept of health, harking back to a primal osteopathic theme but one not entirely in accordance with AT Still's early compatriots.[14]

Analysis

The overall view of the BSO during its first two decades was that of a fragile establishment held together tentatively by JM Littlejohn. He spurned his BOA colleagues' approach of an independent board of controlling trustees. It *is* fortuitous that JM Littlejohn had financial pockets deep enough to provide student loans, many of which were never repaid. Alongside his generosity was his tenacious capacity to fulfil many obligations at the school. For a number of decades the school adopted a low if not defensive profile following its vilification in the Select Committee's Report on Osteopaths (1935). After JM Littlejohn's withdrawal to his beloved study at Badger Hall, his place at the BSO was partially filled by two contenders, the charismatic but mentally volatile Hall and the more modest, dutiful and reflective Webber. They were if anything poles apart, but within these two personalities, the BSO was shaped and personified. Although Webber became principal on JM Littlejohn's death in 1947, Hall never truly accepted this appointment. He resigned from the faculty on a number of occasions until 1964, after which an exasperated Webber never invited him again, but he continued to bluster and provoke from his seat on the BSO board of directors.

Webber maintained a close-knit team of four colleagues plus himself to reorganize and upgrade the course on a more biophysical basis. Much of JM Littlejohn's curriculum and lecture notes were brought up-to-date and the more contentious material was left out until such time that osteopathy found greater acceptance in the general public. There were a large number of osteopaths outside the BSO who were highly critical of these changes but Webber and his team held their nerve for many decades.

References

1. Dove C.I. NOA DVD interview. *Volume 1 – The Early Years*. 2007
2. NOA/T. Edward Hall/File 1 letter to *Time & Tide*. 25th May 1935.
3. Ibid. part 3 correspondence.
4. Hildreth, A.G., *The Lengthening Shadow of Andrew Taylor Still*. Kirksville: Journal Printing. 1938. p.124.
5. Kennard Anne and Sara Littlejohn family interview DVD 2011.
6. Inglis, B., *Fringe Medicine: the case for unorthodox medicine*. London: Faber and Faber. 1964. pp.208–17.
7. Collins, M., p.215.

8. Dove C.I., Conversations. 2007–2010.
9. Collins M., p.227.
10. BMJ, 'Correspondence.' *BMJ*. Vol. No.1. Jan-Jun 3861–3886 (1935): p.967. E. Graham-Little MP.
11. Dove C.I. NOA/CIDove/File1 BSO Curricula 1936–7.
12. Ibid.
13. O'Brien, J.C., 'S. J. Webster-Jones DO MRO.' *British Osteopathic Journal*. Vol. X. 1993. p.5.
14. Dove C.I., NOA DVD Interview. *Cranial Osteopathy*. Vol. 3. 2007.

Chapter 7

The British College of Naturopathy and Osteopathy

Précis

Stanley Lief (1894–1963) emerged as a truly outstanding naturopathic guru. He was a charismatic entrepreneur whose influence resonated throughout the profession. While James Thomson, Edgar Saxon, Harry Clements, Andrew Pitcairn Knowles and Milton Powell laid the foundations of Nature Cure and Naturopathy, it was Stanley Lief who forged a more publicity-aware route through his highly successful Champneys Nature Cure Resort. In 1949, Hector Frazer was particularly impressed by Lief's considerate treatment of his ailing wife. He proposed to endow a building for the peripatetic British College of Naturopathy (BCN). Five years later he opened 'Frazer House' at Netherhall Gardens, Hampstead. Lief, who was ably assisted by his first wife, Stella continued as titular Dean until his death.

In 1961, the college was renamed the British College of Naturopathy and Osteopathy (BCNO) to reflect a close association between the two disciplines and some due deference to osteopathy's greater public profile. Meanwhile, a favourable dialogue had been conducted with the General Council and Register of Osteopaths (GCRO), but simultaneously, the GCRO was proceeding to sue in the High Court a British Naturopathic Association (BNA) practitioner for using the title "Registered Osteopath". Following the outcome of this costly action, the BNA and College changed their name so that alumni could use their designation "Registered Naturopath and Osteopath". In 1964 after Lief's death, a new dean, Albert Rumfitt, was able to establish a full-time course. In the following year Frazer House accommodated the French School of Osteopathy from Paris. BCNO courses were organised from Mondays to Thursdays and the French School met intermittently Fridays to Sundays. Cultural differences in addition to disparities of ethos, training methodology and faculty eventually led to the French School moving to John Wernham's Maidstone Institute in 1971.

Meanwhile, all was not sweetness and light among some radical BCNO students and faculty members who increasingly focussed their attention on the developments in the BCNO which appeared to compare unfavourably with the French, now European, school

69

to reflect an international student body, in Maidstone. Three years later, an irrevocable split took place at the BCNO with two thirds of BCNO students and a quarter of the faculty cutting all ties with their alma mater to train at the newly founded European School Of Osteopathy, Maidstone. In broad terms, a radical element among BCNO staff and students had clashed with a more conservative management resulting in many leaving. This catharsis led to the metamorphosis of a BCNO modelled on sounder scientific basis. Its romantic predecessor was subsumed into a more rational prototype.

Historical Examination

The Nature Cure Association (NCA) had been loosely set up in 1921 but was legally formalised in 1925, probably following its opposition to the British Osteo-pathic Association (BOA) manifesto. NCA antagonism to this was based on the manifesto's claim to exclusive rights to manipulative practice in the UK. For a few years the NCA successfully contained most of the big gurus of natural therapeutics. Then in 1928, James Thomson and his disciples left in high dudgeon at the NCA's inability to set up an adequate school that offered a course similar to Thomson's own full-time, four-year one at the Edinburgh School of Natural Therapeutics (ESNT). On behalf of the NCA, Milton Powell and Harry Clements did attempt to pursue Thomson's ideals and founded such an establishment, the London School of Natural Therapeutics (LSNT) in Kensington. Yet all to no avail as far as Thomson was concerned. He thought the part-time LSNT no substitute for the Edinburgh model. Perhaps the Scottish Thomson feared rivalry from someone south of the border, but he did have a point. Up until then naturopathic education in London had been somewhat haphazard.

One school was established in Ranelagh Gardens and it existed for almost two decades until its closure during the Second World War. In the mid-1930s, an approach had been made to the British School of Osteopathy (BSO) to help run a course. By this time, Littlejohn was a frail man, no longer in a position to assist or of a desire to make such attempts. The LSNT ceased functioning in 1936, making way for a larger NCA institution at Wyndham House, Bryanston Square.[1] Unfor-tunately, an incendiary bomb destroyed the building in the early months of the Second World War and the school ceased operating.[2] During these times, a young naturopath who probably has had the greatest influence on UK Nature Cure emerged as a major spokesman, Stanley Lief.

Stanley Lief, born in 1894 at Corsorka, Russia (now Latvia), was the fourth son of Isaac and Henna Lifschitz. The family had emigrated to South Africa in 1907. Isaac ran a store in Roodepoort, a mining village west of Johannesburg. Stanley was given a basic education in the village before leaving for the USA at 18 years old to train in Natural Therapeutics and Physical Culture under Bernarr Macfadden, and also in Chiropractic at the Chicago National College of Chiropractic. His only sister, Frances (Franny) subsequently attended this chiropractic college too.[3] Macfadden, a grandiose self-publicist, pursued notions of the body beautiful for men and women, a zest for living and implied aspirations of greater sexual fulfilment. Previously he had ventured outside the States to extend his publishing empire to include a London publishing house and in 1909 a health hydro on Brighton seafront which closed at the outbreak of the First World War. Macfadden made furthers trips to Britain establishing the health hydro, Orchard Leigh, in the Chiltern Hills, Buckinghamshire after the war. Lief took over as director, leaving Macfadden to concentrate on his American enterprises. Eventually in 1925, Lief transferred the whole enterprise to Champneys, a much grander building. One Orchard Leigh patient described the set-up thus:

"On arrival at Orchard Leigh, I found the accommodation and treatment room somewhat primitive by Champneys standards, but Stanley Lief impressed me enormously. He was then a comparatively young man with a massive physique and an almost unbelievable amount of energy and enthusiasm."[4]

Lief had fashioned himself partly on Bernarr Macfadden. He attributed his interest in Physical Culture to being a 'sickly child'. He avidly read Macfadden's periodicals in order to help him shape his own modest physique to that of his master. Once he had got to know Macfadden, Lief realised he could not hope to emulate such astonishing bombastic bravura. His personality was similarly different, for Lief was a quiet, reflective person, when compared to Macfadden.[5]

However, what Lief may have forfeited in extroversion, he made up genetically. He came from a highly talented community of Latvian Jewish families who had settled in South Africa, making a formidable mark in the professions, commerce and the arts of that country. Lief exemplified these qualities: he not only ran Champneys successfully, he also founded and edited *Health for All*, a monthly Nature Cure magazine for the general public, he undertook work for the NCA, gave public lectures on Nature Cure and taught naturopathy in the evenings. He was an effective clinician, albeit more of an experimentalist with no scientific background. He emphasised the importance of fasting among other modalities. His manipulation comprised of chiropractic/osteopathic high velocity thrust and his own neuromuscular technique, which was a form of deep digital pressure usually spinally applied – John Wernham called it 'thrashing the soft tissues'. His first wife, Stella, assisted him during these undertakings, continuing to do so even after their divorce and his remarriage. Her only son from the marriage, Charles, a BSO

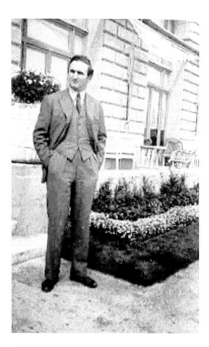

Fig. 19: Stanley Lief as a young man, trying to emulate his mentor, Bernarr Macfadden

graduate, died on the last day of the European campaign of the Second World War.[6] After the end of the war, thoughts and actions over a naturopathic school in London, were revived.

Meanwhile, talks were arranged with the BSO and the British Chiropractic Association (BCA) to launch an integrated school to train all three groups. Principally, the first two years would teach the basic medical sciences, leaving students the penultimate and final years to concentrate on their specific professional practice. None of this appeared to gain consensus with any group, even after further discussion with the BSO. However, in January 1949 the British College of Naturopathy (BCN) was inaugurated.[7]

After a brief peripatetic journey that took in Notting Hill Gate and Lief's flat in Marble Arch, the BCN located to a two-roomed ground floor facility in a narrow terraced house in Craven Gardens, Lancaster Gate, London. Other floors were occupied by ladies of the night. Lief was the titular head accorded to his status, and Dean (philosophy of nature cure and dietetics), Brian Youngs (biology); Clifford

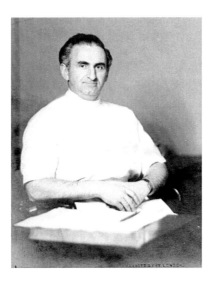

Fig. 20: Stanley Lief in later years

Quick (physics and chemistry); Stella Lief (secretary); Arthur Jenner, responsible for administration and general factotum (anatomy, physiology and physiotherapy) and latterly, Albert Rumfitt (osteopathy).[8] The course contained premedical sciences, the basic medical sciences, dietetics, naturopathy and a smattering of osteopathy with physiotherapy. Lectures took place in the evening when one of the rooms would be converted into a clinic using two screens, which gave three treatment cubicles. The first three intakes consisted of 3–5 students per year paying fees of £100 p.a., who were known by BSO students as 'Lief's Loonies'. Meanwhile, the efforts of a Lief patient, Hector Frazer, had successfully bought a freehold building with formal planning permission given for educational use, in Netherhall Gardens, Hampstead in 1953 for £10,000. A further £5000 was spent on "repairs and alterations".[9]

A year later the BCN was opened with Hector Frazer, Stanley Lief and Albert Rumfitt, President of the British Naturopathic Association (BNA), presiding before a large audience of students and fellow BNA delegates.

The close link between the BCN and BNA continued for some time. In 1959, following Hector Frazer's transfer of the freehold together with a substantial amount of money that matched a similar sum raised by the BNA, the association accepted that a Diploma in Osteopathy (DO) be retracted from them as providers and the BCN instituted its own DO. Coincidentally, the long-standing fracas with

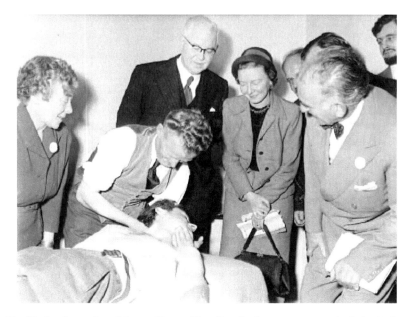

Fig. 21: On the opening of Frazer House. Albert Rumfitt demonstrates a manipulation in front of members of the BNA together with Hector Frazer and Stanley Lief

the General Council and Register of Osteopaths (GCRO) would have an important part to play in the future of the profession.

Tom Moule, another charismatic naturopath, proposed the motion to form a Register of Naturopaths (RGN) and it was carried through. The High Court case brought by the GCRO against a fellow naturopath, WH Dodd, had produced a number of results. The BNA was retitled the British Naturopathic and Osteopathic Association (BNOA) and its members were restricted from using "Registered Osteopath" but could legitimately call themselves "Registered Naturopaths and Osteopaths". The BCN changed to the British College of Naturopathy and Osteopathy (BCNO) and with it the faculty endeavoured to justify the alteration by increasing the osteopathic curriculum. Rumfitt's importance as chief osteopathic lecturer/demonstrator was furthered but Lief's health started to wane.[10]

Above all was a growing awareness that naturopathy was distinctly lesser known than compared with osteopathy and was perhaps even viewed as a bit otherworldly. Naturopathic teaching covered many therapies and it was becoming a bit impractical to discern which to emphasise. Many of the treatments available in a health

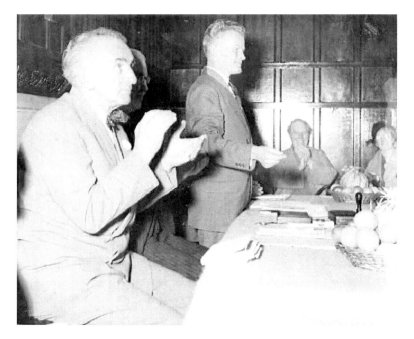

Fig. 22: Albert Rumfitt speaking to BNA members, Hector Frazer and Stanley Lief, nearest

hydro could not be transposed to a private clinic. It was in fact the principles behind naturopathy that had to be emphasised in the curriculum, and these principles lay at the very heart of these diverse 'natural therapies'. It was a mantra for students to learn and pass on to patients – a health code for all. Some colleagues were equally conscious that naturopathic treatment might require time to effect change. In contrast, osteopathic treatment seemed more appealing by providing quicker symptom relief in many cases.[11] Although the Dodd case soured relationships between the GCRO and BNOA for nearly three decades, it laid down a professional and academic commitment to osteopathy. The commitment grew further with the death of Lief in early 1963 and the appointment of Albert Rumfitt as BCNO Dean.

Rumfitt was a pleasant man, opposite in character to the strong Lief. He was never forceful enough, which would have considerable ramifications in time. He forged a bond with John Wernham, no shrinking violet himself, who had waged an acerbic campaign against the BSO, claiming it to be a "third rate medical school". Yet he had incorporated certain naturopathic principles into his daily life. Rumfitt contributed some articles to Wernham's *Maidstone Institute of Applied Technique Year*

Book, in addition to his major contributions to Lief's *Health for All*. Wernham was invited to demonstrate and lecture at the college, capably adamant in proselytising his version of JM Littlejohn's writings. His fervent message matched his personality and at times his manner spilt over, unintentionally or otherwise, at the upset of BCNO students. After much organisation, Rumfitt integrated a full-time Naturopathic and Osteopathic course in 1964, with the college taking on more staff. Some of them were like Wernham, rather robust individuals. Unfortunately, Albert Rumfitt's agreeable style was ineffective in constraining them.[12] Philosophical differences occurred as to whether naturopathic osteopathy should accommodate other adjuncts such as acupuncture and the Alexander Technique.

Bagnall Goodwin, a rational South African Alexander Technique teacher, became BCNO Registrar and general factotum, a responsibility which he conducted fairly efficiently. In addition, he ran the first year course on Naturopathic principles, an eclectic version including Rosicrucian mysticism and other variants. He and his wife, Nancy, occupied the residential flat at Frazer House, which allowed him considerable opportunity to keep well informed, and offered him a unique position to assess the general mood of the student body, faculty and other staff. This situation gave him a valuable perspective with which to advise Albert Rumfitt and the board of governors of any situation arising within its portals. However, Goodwin tended to edit this information to suit himself. Consequently, Rumfitt was never able to quite grasp the important crises that developed over the next decade.[13]

Another BCNO lecturer, Tom Dummer, was to have a major influence not only affecting the BCNO but also determining a wider role for UK osteopathy. Dummer trained as a medical herbalist and taught Naturopathy at the BCNO. He was a charismatic guru, a bon viveur, jazz musician, a quintessentially sociable and non-academic teacher but true green naturopath.[14] His vision of health incorporated a more practical compass of mind, body and soul, utilising a number of other therapies. His approach appeared to oppose the more narrowly interpretative, biophysical concept popular at the time. Perhaps his greatest bonus was to marry a formidable Australian, Margery Warren, who skilfully administered all his professional and domestic activities. Previously she had trained in journalism and public relations and these skills sharpened as she immersed herself in osteopathic matters.[15] A successful institution demands an effective administrator and Margery possessed the levelheadedness to handle an organisation such as the BCNO. Dummer's principles would never have been fulfilled without his wife's common sense, diplomacy, joie de vivre, down-to-earth quality and sheer stamina. Many an osteopathic project has floundered due to poor management and Margery's attention to detail and endeavour prevented many mishaps from developing into irretrievable disasters.

In 1965, the École Française d'Ostéopathie (EFO) in Paris that was training French physiotherapists to combine their expertise with osteopathy seemed to falter. Paul Geny, EFO principal, had been fined many times for practising osteopathy without a state recognised medical degree, this being an essential prerequisite in France. He and the Dummers came to the conclusion that the EFO could be transferred to London. Geny would lecture under Tom's leadership and Margery would be responsible for management and staffing arrangements – no mean feat considering the number of osteopaths involved with messianic tendencies. The BCNO welcomed the EFO (Londres), providing adequate space in Frazer House and its exclusive use for intermittent seminars on a Friday-to-Sunday basis. This arrangement suited all the parties, the BCNO dove-tailed from Mondays to Thursdays, whilst the EFO (Londres) functioned from time to time on the remaining days.

The Dummers had inherited nothing from the school in Paris but 16 stalwart state registered physiotherapists who were willing to travel to London to study osteopathy. Practically, language difficulties were a considerable burden. Few osteopathic books and manuals had been translated into French and few osteopaths apart from Tom could speak fluent French. Fortunately, a bilingual BCNO student, Martine Faure-Alderson came to the rescue. She acted as the official interpreter and transcribed from French to English, a role she continued to perform for many years after graduating. It was agreed that all student fees would be paid to the BCNO, who would reimburse the Dummers by offering them 30% of the takings. All successful students would be duly awarded external BCNO diplomas. Bagnall Goodwin (BCNO registrar) was keen on this arrangement since it relieved the college of much financial worry and provided further use for Frazer House. Tom Dummer assembled an EFO faculty, which reflected some of the best osteopathic technique tutors available. Talented gurus with sizeable egos to match found the school's light atmosphere conducive to their different tasks, and were oblivious to Margery's consummate skills in delivering such an ambiance. News of this exciting venture spread through the grapevine of French physiotherapy and made it a veritably successful proposition.

By 1968, the EFO (Londres) was flourishing and there was a two-year waiting list of French physios wishing to enrol. Overflow seminars were arranged at John Wernham's Maidstone Institute. The increased revenue was welcome in the BCNO's meagre coffers and its osteopathic faculty was further developed. However, dissent started to surface. Some whispered concerns about EFO success in comparison with the BCNO. The two institutions exhibited a different ethos and temperament; a Gallic infectious informality influenced Frazer House, while Goodwin enjoyed the financial rewards of the pact but failed to present a clearer picture of problems arising to Rumfitt and the BCNO governors. Many involved in Frazer House detected an uncomfortable atmosphere of hostility descending through the building. Its existence began to jeopardise the very viability of the EFO (Londres) coexisting under the same roof with its associate college, which was also and importantly its landlord. Goodwin and others did nothing to forestall this gathering situation.[16]

The very nature of osteopathic/naturopathic political wrangling was evolving at the time into a rigid and ossified rancour-suffused relationship. Meanwhile, the BSO was thriving under its new lively principal, Colin Dove, who was developing a four-year course and coordinating a more vigorous campaign to promote student entry. By 1978 the school did have a radical element among its student body but, in 1971–1974 none existed. The GCRO was showing signs of more professionalism and acuity to protect its members by keeping a vigilant eye on those outside its membership using the title "Registered Osteopath". Just to add to the problem, the chilly atmosphere between the BCNO management and the Dummers intensified further.

By 1971, the Dummers had decided to ask Wernham whether it was feasible to move the whole EFO (Londres) organisation to Maidstone. Wernham had a fractious reputation among his colleagues but he readily responded to their wishes. They outlined a European expanded school, École Européene d'Ostéopathie (EEO), fortified by EFO alumni of French speaking Spanish, Swiss, Portuguese and Belgian graduates. More to the point, he enthused over the project by purchasing the house next door, which had recently come on the market. Wernham was made to feel central to their plans and committed at a time when others appeared to shun him and his Littlejohn-led ideals personally. Rigidity is a word that osteopaths use daily in their practices but at this time it exemplified attitudes engendered between osteopathic institutions. The Dummers subsumed Wernham (although he was keen to oblige), but the BCNO's brand appeared to its radical group somewhat backward and sub-mediocre no less.[17] Eventually, the EFO vacated Frazer House, Hampstead, for Tonbridge Road, Maidstone.

The hiatus left by the Dummers, EEO faculty and students had not gone amiss with BNOA staff and students alike. Certainly, the number of students beginning their first year at the BCNO had increased but it appeared that half had been lost by graduation. Nevertheless, the college was growing; indeed more young graduates were joining the faculty. Unfortunately, no one on the board seemed fully to realise that some of its more senior students were becoming politically aware and were critically assessing their naturopathic training. To them, it appeared too formulaic and the osteopathic content ill-conceived and inadequately taught.[18] However, this was not the view of all students, many of whom were quite content to accept the status quo. Meanwhile, the school board was oblivious to these misgivings from the discontent.

The college was structured in a haphazard way. Like all UK osteopathic schools it was staffed by part-timers including the Dean, Albert Rumfitt. The de facto head was Goodwin, a man passionate about his Alexander Technique training but with little knowledge outside that apart from his own eclectic, quasi-philosophical naturopathic interpretation. Goodwin was an elderly man unused or inexperienced in dealing with people voicing a more politically aware agenda. His rather old fashioned, intransigent views were mocked on occasions. For example, he was known to caution students about indulging in acts of making love, announcing that such activity should be considered only sparingly and serve a primarily procreative purpose only. It was as if the 1960's sexual revolution and social upheaval had bypassed him and the college. On the whole, Goodwin, the faculty and British Naturopathic and Osteopathic Association (BNOA) possessed a slightly strange, sanctimonious, self-righteous tone, which dampened students' enquiry and resulted in a less than positive atmosphere. The situation was not helped by the BCNO's attitude towards the International Federation of Practitioners of Natural Therapeutics (IFPNT) following Britain's entry into the Common Market in 1973.

It was advised that the largest British natural therapeutic college should liaise with similar German statutory regulated institutions to quantify educational standards. The BNCO feared that the European Commission might impose the German statutory model on all member countries. In May 1973, at the BNOA annual general meeting, a motion was passed in favour of the BCNO joining the IFPNT to augment European fraternal natural therapeutic cooperation. The school board informed the BNOA that IFPNT membership "was not in the best interests of the BCNO". Consequently, the BNOA committee conveyed this to its membership at an extraordinary general meeting, which carried a motion of dismay, voicing no confidence in the Board.[19] The IFPNT was organised by Tom and Margery Dummers. Perhaps an existing enmity between them and the BCNO had fouled any mutual cooperation, even one fostering intercollegiate facilitations. Such an action was quite alien to other British osteopathic schools too. What appeared to the BCNO board as a reasonable decision had other ramifications beyond BNOA disapproval. Some were young BCNO faculty members and students concerned at the board's apparent disregard of future European regulations. This apprehension spilt over in the college ethos. Where was it leading?

Surprisingly, Wernham was still teaching at the BCNO and this had a positive effect on radical students. Wernham had formed a close professional and social association with Hall. Many of their ideas on osteopathy had emanated from a mutual consideration of JM Littlejohn's influence. They constructed a philosophy and practice based on the twin pillars of JM Littlejohn's writings and Hall's osteopathic technique. Wernham had no compunction in dismissing the efforts of BCNO osteopathic technique lecturers. He seemed insensitive to them. His fractious, damaging message conveyed to students was partly a proselytising version of JM Littlejohn, outmoded from osteopathic mainstream teaching at the time. Together with general criticisms of the course, his rallying to the Maidstone cause played a major part of disaffection among radical students.

Wernham's concept clashed with BCNO hierarchical opinion. He complained about a dearth of academic, technical and clinical osteopathic input at the BCNO. Others alleged that the college performed cosily in a sort of pioneering mode but with little enthusiasm and ambition. To them the naturopathic clinical training appeared too prescriptive, a combination of hydrotherapy, "Nuts 'n' Raisins" diet and Lief's neuromuscular technique. It has been asserted that some were delegated only one patient per week because of poor numbers. Student frustration was based on the clinical formulaic naturopathy and deficient patient experience.[20]

Osteopathy was given lip service but it was alleged that these limitations were exposed in its underprovided library and insufficient teaching. The college ethos expressed by Lief and others had become a melee. Was osteopathy in fact a naturopathic adjunct among many others? Or was it a separate entity with its own set of values, principles and practice? The BCNO had come to a familiar crossroads experienced by all osteopathic schools in considering how to evolve. Osteopathy needed reasoned, empathetic leadership, but in Rumfitt and Goodwin, however decent they might have been, these qualities were not apparent. In 1973, the BCNO contained a number of bright, young, politically motivated faculty members who wished to upgrade the course, uneasy at its lack of inspiration and guidance. Some intelligent students were quite content to see out their days until graduation even though their radically aware colleagues fidgeted uneasily. They perceived an ossified college somewhat at odds with their views. What happened next would have decisive repercussions.[21]

The cohort of younger faculty included Stephen Pirie, Robert Lever, Robin Kirk and Paul Greenhouse, members who were eager to improve standards, uneasy to accept the status quo and keen to equip the profession with a better, more coherent voice. They asked Goodwin to extend the course to include Fridays now that the French school had vacated Frazer House. The request fell on deaf ears. Goodwin replied that Fridays were out of the question as it was cleaning day. Such fatuous remarks led to a feeling that any positive change was unlikely to occur in the foreseeable future. They laid remaining ideas aside and decided to join the Dummers.[22]

The student body was keen to know more about this departure and Rumfitt as dean faced a student meeting that had been arranged to clear the air. Ron Cook asked the obvious question. Why were young members of the faculty resigning? An exasperated Rumfitt flew into a rage and refused to answer the question, suggesting instead that they all got on with their studies. A few days later, Goodwin placed an ultimatum on the college notice board to the effect that any further unwarranted discussions on this subject would lead to instant dismissal. Rumfitt had been poorly informed all along. Students did not want to jeopardise their BCNO training but they did want an explanation as to why the governors were remaining inflexible to younger facultys' demands for change. When their aspirations were ignored they decided to resign and follow the Dummers. If Goodwin thought that this escalation would bring the student body to its senses, he had another thing coming.

Martin Booth organised a series of ex-officio student meetings to be held away from Frazer House with individual faculty members to find out their reasons for leaving. From these, Martin Booth and Harold Klug were delegated to arrange a meeting with the BCNO board of governors to consider their concerns. Goodwin was unhelpful, replying that such a meeting was impractical, declaring he could not hope to obtain a quorum of the board at such short notice.

The very next weekend, Martin Booth found there was a gathering and duly wrote down the number plates displayed in the car park of those attending the board meeting. On hearing this, the student body felt that they had been deceived; Goodwin had been economical with the truth. Conversation centred on whether students could transfer to Maidstone to join their teachers. Meanwhile, Harold Klug was assigned to talk to Tom Dummer about their predicament.[23] A few days later, Klug initiated another meeting with the Dummers to see whether students could transfer to a new school in Maidstone. Margery gave the go-ahead for BCNO students to enrol in the newly formed European School of Osteopathy (ESO) under her management at the Wernham Institute, 28–30 Tonbridge Road, Maidstone, in four month's time. During discussion at a gathering of students, two thirds elected to transfer to the ESO to form a second, third and fourth year, Barry Lonergan joined the BSO, and the rump remained.[24]

As a postscript, Harold Klug, Barry Lonergan and Martin Booth were invited to attend a BNOA meeting at Frazer House attended by 50 interested members. They informed everyone. There was never any intention by the student body to leave the BCNO but it was refused any meeting with the college board and reiterated the spurious reason given for denying such a request. Martin Booth provided evidence of car number plates present in the car park and of those board members attending during the following Saturday's governors' meeting. People present were uncomfortable and quite mystified at the Board's behaviour. Thus the revolution was not a deliberate event but an accidental result of circumstance.

Analysis

This episode highlights a number of events including social upheaval where radical and reactionary consequences collided to cause disarray, even among already splintered osteopathic groups. Student disaffection in the late 1960s had culminated in student unrest at their respective UK colleges and universities. Mysteriously, this found resonance among a number of BCNO students, which was surprising considering the rather conservative nature of all osteopathic schools. Goodwin, de facto principal, behaving as an authoritarian septuagenarian of right-wing political views, exacerbated this. He was a decent but intransigent fellow. He and his wife, Nancy, appeared as despots, disposing favour and authority in variable amounts. Rumfitt and his deputy dean, Denis Kiely, taught osteopathic technique and allied subjects reasonably, giving them their best shot. However, they and others were being undermined by Wernham, whose JM Littlejohn-interpreted version he considered the gold standard. Pivotal to this was a cohort of radical BCNO third year students, some of which had retained links with Dummer and Wernham outside the BCNO.

The festering climate was heightened by all osteopathic schools being dependent upon the services of altruistic lecturers and tutors willing to give their cherished time for a pittance. These institutions had been haphazardly run at the best of times, which made them appear rather aimless and sluggish. Osteopaths, like many others, do not make natural public speakers and the content of their lectures can be somewhat woolly too. Indeed, it was the junior members of the faculty that clamoured for change in the first place. Some of the more inflexible old guard appeared out of touch, treating young staff and students like some sergeant major or officious trade unionist.[25] Although many students could understand this amateurish ethos it did nothing to appease the more radically inclined, especially during these restless times.

Goodwin, an ex-banker, who quintessentially observed BCNO matters in financial terms, exacerbated the situation. More importantly, his authoritarian manner grievously underestimated a desire by some staff and students for him and Rumfitt to explain BCNO management's intransigence. Suddenly, Rumfitt and Goodwin misconstrued events, making their intentions appear devious and shoddy, which resulted in a quarter of staff and two thirds of students departing to join the newly established European School of Osteopathy in Maidstone. The struggle to maintain the status quo is reminiscent of episodes in earlier osteopathic history, including that of AT Still versus the Littlejohn brothers and Bill Smith at Kirksville in 1900. No doubt Tom Dummer and John Wernham were far stronger characters for college governors to contend with but they were the beneficiaries of an exceptional cohort of young faculty and ex-BCNO students.[26] Whether those more radical among staff and students could have been appeased is mere conjecture. Could Goodwin's resignation have alleviated some of the situation? One doubts it. Could Rumfitt, part-time dean, have achieved more credence among them? Probably not. Goodwin, shocked by their departure, became the fall guy, a forlorn figure out of his depth and struggling to convey misplaced authority. He never regained his composure and died relatively soon afterwards.

In September 1976, Denis Kiely became BCNO dean, Ian Drysdale his deputy and full-time lecturer. From this catharsis, the BCNO emerged to evolve its curriculum on a more scientific basis but within a more osteopathic appreciation rather than a naturopathic one to bring about the British College of Osteopathic Medicine.

References

1. Chambers, M.M., *The British Naturopathic Association – the First Fifty Years.* Sevenoaks, Kent: The British Naturopathic Association. 1996. pp.7–9; p.11.
2. Collins, M., *Osteopathy in Britain: the first hundred years.* London: Booksurge. 2005. pp.179–80.
3. Stanley and Peter Lief family archive held at NOA. Letters from Stanley W Lief and Boris Chaitow.
4. Ibid. Letter from Colonel Bunbury.
5. Lowe Ken, NOA DVD Interview. 2011.
6. Youngs Brian K., NOA DVD Interview. 2009.
7. Chambers M., pp.10–1; p.15.
8. Youngs B.K.
9. Kiely D., NOA DVD Interview. 2007.
10. Chambers M., pp.15 -25.
11. Newman Turner, R., NOA DVD Interview. 2010.
12. Kiely, D., Interview.

13. Kirk, Robin, NOA DVD Interview. 2008.
14. Youngs, B.K., Interview.
15. Bloomfield, M., *Tree of Life*. Brighton: Indepenpress. 2009. p.xiii.
16. Ibid pp.9–19.
17. Ibid pp.9–19.
18. Lever, Robert., NOA DVD Interview. 2008.
19. Bloomfield, M., pp.26–7.
20. Booth, Martin, Phone interview. 22nd June 2011.
21. Lever, R., Interview.
22. Kirk, R., Interview.
23. Klug, Harold NOA DVD Interview. 2009.
24. Lonergan, Barry interview by phone 12th July 2011. Three third year students remained and second years remained, bar three who left for the ESO and Barry Lonergan to the BSO. Barry gave his reason for leaving; Ian Drysdale's resignation from the faculty in April. Had he known that Ian was to return that autumn he would not have transferred to the BSO.
25. Kirk, R., Interview.
26. Kiely, D., Interview.

Chapter 8

Heading Towards Professional Unity

Précis

The breakaway of osteopathy from the British College of Naturopathy and Osteopathy (BCNO) and formation of the European School of Osteopathy (ESO) at John Wernham's Institute was a triumph of expectation over financial expediency. Here, Wernham was able to expound his version of JM Littlejohn's principles, practice and his General Osteopathic Treatment (GOT) while Tom Dummer and others were able to develop Parnell Bradbury's hypothesis of Specific Adjustment Technique (SAT). Eventually, GOT and SAT adherents polarised into two camps culminating in the ESO.

This action brought about a flowering of SAT, purporting to convert the British School of Osteopathy's (BSO) biopathophysical model into a more universal concept. Call it naïve or almost evangelical, but it acted as a clarion call for those frustrated within a clinical rut of minor orthopaedic conditions. Among the fringes of osteopathic practice was a further counterclaim from cranial practitioners. Colin Dove had been sent on a mission to the Sutherland Cranial Teaching Foundation (SCTF) in the USA to verify its worth but he returned fortified to learn more. Meanwhile, the apolitical Society of Osteopaths (SO) had been set up for ESO alumni, ex-BCNO alumni and travelling osteopaths to disseminate the ESO ethos, principles and practice to a wider audience, encourage non-competitive relationships respectful of other rival institutions and to further professional unity.

Hitherto, Dove had been appointed Associate Board Member of the SCTF that had awarded medical practitioners, dentists and General Council and Register of Osteopaths (GCRO) members' eligibility rights to attend SCTF courses. Rollin Becker, SCTF president, granted Dove permission to extend this agreement to SO associates, although he never ratified this with his full Board. This mutual trust resulted in SO members joining the BSO cranial foundation. Independently, the British College of Naturopathy and Osteopathy (BCNO) had linked up with fellow SCTF member, John Upledger, to teach cranial therapy at Frazer House.

From these visits, Upledger had been informed of the disunity among UK osteopaths and the role the GCRO appeared to play in maintaining this status quo. This supposedly vitriolic situation was conveyed by Upledger to the presidents of the Applied Academy of Osteopaths (AAO), the American Osteopathic Association (AOA) and delegates at an AAO convention attended by Dove. Afterwards, Edna Lay, a formidable Californian practitioner, arranged a meeting between Upledger and Dove.

Under the auspices of an SO symposium, Dove and Upledger met Dummer and an inner circle of SO confidants to outline a scheme for ESO accreditation and enabling SO members to join the GCRO en bloc. After many months of bargaining, ESO alumni and SO members were eligible to collectively join the GCRO. Their representatives, John Barkworth and Simon Fielding, were invited on to an intimidating GCRO council. SO entry facilitated BCNO graduates to follow suit four years later. Undoubtedly, the catalyst for unification was Dove. His meetings with fellow adherents from the BSO, ESO, BCNO and American SCTF officials brought about this long-awaited break-through beneath a broader professional umbrella of a genuine desire to unify the profession.

Historical Examination

The first five years of the European School of Osteopathy (ESO) and its sister college, the École Européene d'Ostéopathie (EEO) established three years before, was spent at John Wernham's Maidstone Institute of Applied Technique at 28–30 Tonbridge Road. The ex-BCNO third year students made up the final year ESO cohort. They were an exceptional bunch.[1] Margery Dummer continued to balance the constraints of finance with subtle diplomacy, managing to keep everyone happy. Many students had lost their local government grants following their BCNO departure and as a result, an atmosphere of make do and extemporise pervaded the building during those early days.

John Wernham was delighted to have such a willing captive audience to explain his version of the Littlejohn osteopathy and his General Osteopathic Treatment (GOT) to. Wernham's physical stature coupled with his booming voice, deliberately annunciating each syllable of every word, provided a visual and aural spectacle. GOT was interpreted as reducing spinal dysfunctions so as to mould the body to respond within healthy bounds, allowing it to function more efficiently.

Although Wernham was respectful of Tom Dummer's aims, he could not quite accept the principles behind his Specific Adjustment Technique (SAT). Dummer had evolved this from Parnell Bradbury's more rudimentary notion, based on an amalgam of chiropractic and osteopathic theory and practice. Dummer's perspective of body, mind and soul was not intended for an ethereal audience but instead as a plea for openness, kindling a new osteopathic order. SAT was a subtle resource and the least invasive procedure, unlocking or releasing tissues or energy through harnessing the healing powers of the body. SAT cognisance was the ability to find the switch which turns on this power. In contrast, the BSO's biopathophysical concept of health endeavoured to differentiate tissues and their condition involved in somatic dysfunction.

Dummer wished, perhaps unconsciously, to return to Still's magnetic healing, phrenomagnetic experiences, notions of which were misinterpreted until Sutherland's cranial hypothesis was given some credence.[2] Specific Adjustment Technique (SAT) was formulated by Parnell Bradbury, a practitioner trained as an osteopath and chiropractor who worked closely with Dummer. It started from the body's own lack of response to inside and outside stimuli and considered how treatment could provide resources to overcome this problem and which techniques should enhance this action. GOT appeared to work from the opposite end of the healing spectrum. SAT was courageous, eclectic, evangelical and naïve but nectar to avid students who were thirsting for knowledge. Although it was very 'Littlejohn' in content, Wernham did not believe this to be the case. Even Margery's powers of peacekeeping and tact could no longer save the deteriorating relationship between Wernham and the ESO, although her public decorum seldom disappeared.

Wernham was becoming more abrasive and derogatory of the ESO's SAT ethos, polarising people into two camps. Overwhelmingly, ESO students sided with Dummer and his hypothesis. Personal criticism made the process of departure inevitable and more rapid. To his credit, Wernham raised the money for the ESO to move to 104 Tonbridge Road and continued to provide clinic cover for its students down the road at his Institute. He displayed instances of great kindness such as these, but they were unfortunately neutralised at times by his incompatible and forceful behaviour. Meanwhile, Tom Dummer had started to develop his thoughts and actions around an inner circle of confidants, organising his Society of Osteopaths (SO) based on membership from ESO alumni, ex-BCNO graduates and other self-respecting osteopaths.

Robert Lever and Harold Klug had been appointed by Dummer to organise and edit a regular journal and arrange SO symposia and events. Dummer was prone to becoming exasperated and despairing at the various antics of his profession but Lever advised him to take logical steps in developing programmes and subject matter to keep a balanced perspective, advocating caution rather than invective.[3] Lever realised that there was enough maverick behaviour outside ESO confines without more being added to it. Unbeknown to his colleagues, Dummer had maintained a regular correspondence with Colin Dove (BSO principal 1968–76),

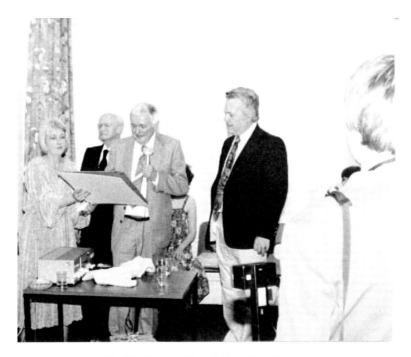

Fig. 23: Margery Bloomfield and Tom Dummer

who had much sympathy with his plight.[4] Dummer also recognised Dove's strength in straight talking without malice or personal denigration.

Lever and Klug recognised that these were heady days. The question now was how they could address fossilised enmity and mistrust among osteopathic institutions, regulatory bodies and associations. As they were only too aware of their own experiences at the BCNO and Maidstone Institute, situations could rapidly deteriorate by developing into irrevocable schisms.

Lever and Klug had a genuine, almost evangelical desire to extol the virtues of expanding osteopathic concepts and broaden their basis. Yet many osteopathic groups would try to score points off each other in *Medical News* and other organs, much to the delight of the profession's enemies. Lever and Klug's policy was to ignore enmity, division and disparagements within the profession, treating them as if they did not exist and instead dealing with all colleagues with respect, equality and amity.[5] It was no simple task. Where was there an empathetic group of like-minded osteopaths willing to form loose alliances? Yet it was not difficult to acknowledge one innovative group of BSO graduates who appreciated the subtler

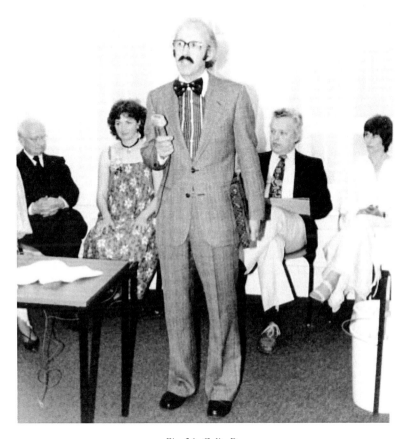

Fig. 24: Colin Dove

cranial concept that had been expounded by William Sutherland decades before at the expense of a more mechanistic model.

Still had experienced much sustenance from magnetic healing during and after the American Civil War found interest in "ideas of the central tenets" and "health as the harmonious interaction of all the body's parts and the unobstructed flow of fluid".[6] He would have been astutely aware of other alternative movements like phrenology. Phrenomagnetism appeared to give the soul a form of 'spiritual energy', very much connected to the brain and spinal cord, and life itself. As one phrenomagnetist stated "without magnetism phrenology is no more than a body without a soul. For what is a brain or its developments, without life?"[7]

Sutherland had developed ideas very similar to phrenomagnetism. Although his interpretation was somewhat mechanistic too, his hypothesis continued to evolve and flourish within the US Cranial Academy of Osteopathy and Sutherland Cranial Teaching Foundation (SCTF). Various American cranial practitioners held courses in Paris and London introducing his principles and practice to different schools and associations. Eddie Gilhooley was the first exponent in this country, learning from Sutherland himself. Gilhooley went on to teach Denis Brookes, a good friend of Dummer's and a fellow EFO faculty member.[8] The cranial concept became a conduit for osteopathic change, not only in a practice sense but also politically. Lever and Klug saw a means to evolve SO activities through contact with cranial devotees from the British School of Osteopathy (BSO) alumni.

Jack Taylor was brought into the SO close circle, equally disliking all formal committee dealings. His personality seemed to complement that of Klug and Lever. He was quiet and affable, efficiently handling paperwork with osteopathic contacts outside his own graduate colleagues. Through this he was able to facilitate the whole process of setting up a network of cranial adherents. One must remember that the cranial model was perceived by many osteopaths as other-worldly and this pioneering spirit gave the minority group further ground for empathising with supporters from dissimilar training backgrounds. Two BSO graduates, Stuart Korth and Joyce Vetterlein, fell into this category, providing useful links to forge with them an informal network.[9]

Colin Dove, meanwhile, had been given a financial grant by the BSO board of governors to attend an American SCTF symposium in order to ascertain the worth of the cranial notion. All official ties with UK-trained osteopaths had been irrevocably cut in 1925, yet here were their US counterparts, not only welcoming them as colleagues but also travelling to Europe to teach them. Dove returned to Britain to inform his Board that the venture had been fruitful. In fact, it led to him becoming a devotee. He organised future regular BSO cranial training sessions under the auspices of the US SCTF using their tutors and lecturers and he was made an associate board member of the SCTF. Taylor, Klug and Lever deduced from Korth and Vetterlein that Dove could provide a realistic opportunity towards achieving unity within osteopathy.

By now, Dove had already been BSO principal for eight years and he was prepared to continue in that position but the BSO governors decided to appoint a new principal with greater academic experience. Throughout his tenure, Dove's energy had been irrepressible and his leadership refreshing, marked by a forthright, pragmatic attitude. If he thought an idea would not work, he was not afraid to share his beliefs regardless of who he was talking to. He accepted the Board's decision and instead turned his attention towards cranial education by cementing further connections with the SCTF, BSO cranial courses and, significantly, becoming vice-chairman of the GCRO. He continued to develop his long-standing friendship with Dummer, who was respectful of Dove's reputation for realistically assessing problems and tactfully dismissing unfeasible proposals. Above all else, Dummer and his SO triumvirate trusted him. Dove set about innovating subtle changes, laying the foundations for stepping stones towards unity.

The SCTF had agreed to teach three groups: physicians; dentists; and GCRO registered osteopaths. Dove approached the august SCTF president, Rollin Becker, asking him to allow SO members to join the BSO cohort of members as honorary GCRO members in anticipation of their intended GCRO enrolment. Becker trusted Dove's judgement, not only acceding to his request but also giving him free rein to bring in other alumni whose institutions were negotiating to join the GCRO. However, unbeknown to Dove, Becker never took the matter to his board for ratification and this omission would backfire with bitter consequences a decade later.

Meanwhile, one of the SO group, Susan Turner, became the first non-GCRO member of the BSO cranial faculty to emerge as one of the finest cranial teachers throughout the world.[10] Another American SCTF member, John Upledger, had been championed by the BCNO, and had been teaching a cranial course at Frazer House. He was conscious of BCNO antipathy towards the GCRO, which purportedly ran a closed shop excluding many from joining. At an American Applied Academy of Osteopathy (AAO) convention, he outlined this supposed injustice to members. Fortunately, Dove was attending the very same meeting and agreed to attend a private hearing with the presidents of the AAO and American Osteopathic Association (AOA), the formidable Californian osteopath Edna Lay and John Upledger.

Dove was able to allay fears that the GCRO was operating a closed shop, intimating instead an aspiration from the GCRO council for all colleges to apply to join the umbrella organization. With Upledger's help Dove claimed that this goal could become a reality. They both had been invited to speak at a forthcoming SO symposium. Upledger had apparently already formed convivial relations with SO officials including Harold Klug and his wife, Naomi. Individuals such as Irwin Korr, former head of research at Kirksville, Missouri, became good friends and were very sympathetic towards UK osteopathy,[11] which was significant because there had been no formal links between the American Osteopathic Association and British-trained osteopaths since 1926. It was hoped that a newly optimistic atmosphere was gradually leading to greater respect among the UK antagonist groups, and the result would be a move towards compromise.

The SO trio decided to ask the Osteopathic Association of Great Britain (OAGB), the BSO alumni organisation, whether SO members were eligible to join. At an OAGB annual general meeting it was favourably moved to accept SO individual membership. However, Barry Savory, a BSO graduate and President of the SO, was more cautious, stating that it was better to remain independent from the OAGB rather than incur GCRO wrath. After a particularly successful day at the duly selected SO symposium, Tom Dummer, Margery Bloomfield, Robert Lever, Harold Klug, Simon Fielding, Colin Dove and John Upledger met in the ESO flat at 104 Tonbridge Road, Maidstone, to devise a course of action.[12]

Upledger harangued the group about the desperate state of UK osteopathic politics, leaving all present with no lingering doubt as to where his sympathies lay. Dove interposed a novel solution. He suggested his BSO cranial faculty could allow SO members to enrol on courses, giving them identical rights to GCRO osteopaths. He proposed arranging a GCRO/SO joint meeting to discuss a process for the SO to register with the GCRO en bloc. He suggested the ESO apply *informally* to a school inspection by a GCRO team. Recommendations from its report would then be implemented by the ESO. After this the ESO could formally request a GCRO inspection and all things being equal, accreditation and eligibility en masse for SO members to join the GCRO would be accepted.[13] The question now was how would the GCRO react to these propositions?

Since 1978, the GCRO had been working towards some sort of accommodation with opposing groups. Michael van Straten (BNOA), Denis Kiely (BNOA) and Douglas Drysdale (President of the BNOA) met up with a GCRO deputation including Vice-Chairman Dove to discuss mutual concerns. All agreed that this war of attrition over the title "Registered Osteopath" could not be defended in High Court by either party and would leave both bankrupt. GCRO representatives requested the BNOA restrain four individual members from using the title. Everyone knew that realistically, the GCRO could not police or sue anyone for displaying the title "Registered Osteopath". It could only implement an illegal use of the letters MRO (Member of the Register of Osteopaths). Also discussed was an independent inspection of the BCNO and BSO by a team of neutral educationalists to ascertain the worth of each.[14] These discussions, however useful, were rather set aside by the determined efforts of some GCRO officials and their SO counterparts to procure GCRO accreditation and SO membership to the Register.

Len Nugent (GCRO Chairman), Colin Dove (Vice-Chairman) and Barrie Dare-wski (GCRO Secretary) met up with SO executives, Harold Klug, Robert Lever and Simon Fielding, to discuss logistics for ESO accreditation and the SO to enrol onto the GCRO en bloc. It was agreed to follow the procedure that Dove had previously outlined. John Barkworth (SO) would negotiate terms and memoranda with Maurice Hills (GCRO Registrar) and Harold Klug (ESO) would confer with Greg Sharp (GCRO Education). It was a tortuous, gruelling process requiring tact, stamina, goodwill and mutual understanding. Yet over numerous phone calls and meetings the process was finally ratified after 20 months.[15] This led to a successful resolution with SO members, John Barkworth and Simon Fielding, who under some reluctance joined an intimidating GCRO council. In time both flourished, becoming outstanding officials and further contributing to an ever-increasing GCRO professionalism.

Analysis

After many decades of internecine struggles, a realisation was taking place throughout the profession that changes were required to in order to accommodate all osteopaths. How that would occur was problematical and circumspect. However, it was the development of a more biopsychosocial model that brought about this thaw. Cranial concept fulfilled much of this new role. It was already advanced among a small group of US osteopathic physicians who taught on visits to Europe. Some semi-official recognition from these US colleagues towards their European counterparts opened a considerable rapprochement, which had been denied since 1926.

Colin Dove had a substantial influence over these proceedings. He was a keen cranial exponent, an associate SCTF board member who also ran the BSO cranial courses and was GCRO vice-chairman. He played a pivotal role in reviewing the SO's successful application and ESO accreditation. Equally, the roles of Harold Klug, Robert Lever, Jack Taylor, latterly Simon Fielding and John Barkworth for the SO were decisive. Moreover, Michael van Straten (BNOA) and his colleagues showed an understanding of difficulties arising between the two groups. The GCRO welcomed the climate of change and tolerance. It was reassuring to realise that collectively, osteopaths could negotiate through their different backgrounds to acknowledge how much they had in common. Many decades of fruitless indifference and hostility, wasted energy and money, was all grist to the mill. As the Bob Dylan song ascribed, "The times they are a-changin."

References

1. Barkworth, John, NOA DVD Interview. 2009.
2. Lever, Robert, NOA DVD Interview. 2008.
3. Klug, Harold, NOA DVD Interview. 2009.
4. Dove, Colin., I NOA DVD Vol. 3. Cranial Interview. 2008. NOA *Colin Dove archive/* Vol. 3/letters from T. Dummer.
5. Klug, H., *Interview*.
6. Gevitz, N., *The DOs*. Baltimore: John Hopkins University Press. 1982. pp.12–14.
7. Fuller, R.C., *Mesmerism and the American Cure of Souls*. Philadelphia: University of Pennsylvania Press. 1982. p.53.
8. NOA Cranial section, CRA/Files 1–5: Sutherland; CRA/File 5 Denis Brookes' letter.
9. Klug, H., Interview.
10. Dove C.I., NOA DVD Vol. 3. Cranial Interview.
11. Klug H. Interview.
12. Ibid.
13. Dove C.I., Interview.
14. NOA/GCRO/CO/Minutes/File 3: 6-09-1978 p.3; 14-01-1979; 5-12-1980 p.1; 9-02-1981 p.1.
15. Ibid: 3-04-1981 p.1; 9-02-82; 7-03-1982; 30-04-1982; 7–061982; 20-09-1982; 21-12-1982.

Chapter 9

Osteopathy Comes of Age: Legislation and the General Osteopathic Council

Précis

The General Council and Register of Osteopaths (GCRO) moved steadily forward under its secretary, Barrie Darewski. It remained very much part of the British School of Osteopathy (BSO), if not in spirit certainly in body. Darewski ran the growing organisation on a shoestring. In time, Lieutenant-Colonel Peter Blaker succeeded him as GCRO secretary. Another council member offered this advice: "you must be mad to take on this; watch your back; and they are a bit of a shower".[1] It was not an ideal start in a world according to Jocelyn Proby of "frightfully lower middle-class" osteopaths.

Very few others involved in UK osteopathy have had Blaker's vision. He restructured the GCRO into an outfit for well-intentioned, emerging professionals. Once it was established that the voluntary GCRO was professionally organised, procedure moved on to include the whole profession. In 1986, Nigel Clarke provided the strategy not only to overcome numerous hurdles but the entrée and ability to do so. Clarke offered valuable support to the latest GCRO chairman, Simon Fielding, to develop his persona further and he became a consummate osteopathic politician. Meanwhile, Harold Klug and Robert Lever provided the wherewithal for change. Fielding's parliamentary networking continued at a pace.

Finally, Robyn Balderstone secured assistance from Lord Skelmersdale to draught four key points to the proposals: upgrading education standards to conform to those of other state regulated healthcare professions; agreeing acceptable ethical ideals; achieving unity of purpose within the osteopathic profession; and finding the support of the medical profession. It was a daunting task. The GCRO council was passive to the process, fearing failure of the project, causing further retribution from a hostile medical establishment; considerable vitriol and mistrust from non-GCRO osteopaths; and no cooperation from government or medical sources. Over and above this, no alternative group had successfully sought approval since homeopathic physicians through royal patronage in the Medical Act (1858).

*It was Skelmersdale that introduced Fielding and Clarke to one of the Prince of Wales'
confidants, Lord Kindersley, and the Prince provided help from that time on. The King's
Fund feasibility enquiry on osteopathic statutory regulation was under the effective
control of Sir Thomas Bingham. Jane Langer and John Armitstead played important
roles in the process. Within a few meetings, any animosity disappeared between the
osteopathic representatives and the three medical ones, Ian Todd, Sir John Walton and
David Shaw. From that time, Bingham was able to chair a committee willing to draught
a blueprint for successful conclusion, through Parliament, towards statutory regulation
and Royal Assent in 1993.*

Historical Examination

Barrie Darewski was an affable man with a capacity for getting along with most
people. His great friend Lord Cullen of Ashbourne, Chairman of the GCRO and
the Osteopathic Education Foundation (OEF), had introduced Darewski to the
GCRO council as a suitable replacement for Michael Morris. Darewski had been an
excellent cricketer. He understood only too well the machinations of the antiquated
Marylebone Cricket Club, the intricacy of the rules of the game and oddness of
some players. These attributes were to help him deal with the eccentricities of
individual osteopaths. Fortunately he was endowed with a good sense of humour
and general bonhomie. At times he could be wary of his osteopathic fraternity and
sorority outside the GCRO camp, once claiming, "If you lay down with dogs,
expect to get fleas." By and large he was a peacemaker and a useful person to have
at the helm during lengthy negotiations with the ESO and Society of Osteopaths
(SO), later the British College of Naturopathy and Osteopathy (BCNO) and
British Naturopathic and Osteopathic Association (BNOA).

Darewski ran the GCRO office with the help of one other person, reputedly
subsidising her from his own pocket. His office was located in the BSO cellars at
Buckingham Gate until the school transferred to its grandiose building off
Trafalgar Square. The GCRO was reputed to be an appendage of the BSO and its
location and sharing of secretarial staff supported this opinion. The GCRO council
could have reflected this view but fortunately a more open-minded ethos existed to
benefit other groups in the forms of Dr Patterson (London College of Osteopathic
Medicine), Simon Fielding and John Barkworth (ESO/SO). At the end of
Darewski's tenure as GCRO secretary he was awarded an OBE for services to the
profession, and was fondly remembered as a good man.

After Darewski's departure Lieutenant-Colonel Peter Blaker took over as secretary.
In contrast he was a man with conflicting personality traits. He was educated at
Lancing College and St John's, Cambridge, before joining the army for his

National Service. On its completion he converted a regular commission. Blaker spent 22 years in the services, cutting short an extension to retire due to illness. He entered into his GCRO work with gusto. His intention was to place the GCRO on a firm, sound professional footing and to proceed towards statutory regulation.

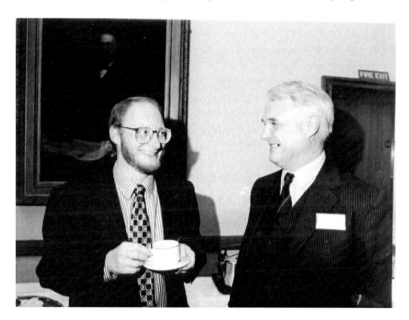

Fig. 25: Simon Fielding and Peter Blaker at the New Cavendish Club

Blaker's first thought was that the profession consisted of a group with limited horizons. However, he was acutely aware of its members' dedicated, kind, thought-fulness and empathy towards their patients. At the same time, the GCRO council was going round in circles whilst battling with infighting. They appeared to be frightened of change and had turned into an insubstantial set-up that was poorly administered. Blaker became quite frustrated by the council's inability to set boundaries. During his military experience he had been able to work effectively within some confines. Yet now he felt unable to carry out his responsibilities and report back to the council without creating some friction. To counter this problem his standards were stringent. He insisted that the GCRO council meetings should be adequately staffed with a proper agenda and supporting papers, administration should be efficiently run, accounts undertaken following correct procedure and documentation was to be clearer and professionally written to fit osteopathy's new standing.[2] These aspirations were all well and good but could he carry out such a formidable task without ruffling too many feathers? He had the capabilities to carry out such reform and the intelligence to do so. But did he have the temperament to take the council and membership with him?

His GCRO council had a number of noteworthy individuals. The Chairman, Barry Lambert, was a man of honour and integrity although perhaps at times a little hesitant. He had held the council together during these reforms. Lambert was a good public speaker, one who might be described as 'a safe pair of hands'. His Registrar, Maurice Hills, had integrity and ability, was waspish but also straightforward. Simon Fielding, parliamentary activities, was able, charming, humorous and great fun and John Barkworth had, perhaps, the quickest brain and was very caring. Others too went along with these improvements.[3] Blaker obtained permission to transfer the GCRO offices to Reading near to his home, although council meetings and Annual General Meetings remained in London. It was a good move because it spiked the notion of it being a BSO institution. From the new London Street premises his reorganised administrative centre took on more staff and further responsibilities. His successful accomplishments came at a price and his impatience and fastidious demeanour could erupt at times. Simon Fielding had been given free rein by Lambert to undertake general political enquiry into statutory regulation.

One of his first parliamentary contacts was Tony Durant MP, a friend of Bob and Margery Bloomfield (ex-Dummer). In truth his professional family was the Osteopathic Genesis Foundation (OGF) colleagues and a few ESO contacts sustained his passion for statutory regulation. Yet it was one thing to extol its virtues among friends and family at social functions but it was another to repeatedly bring the matter up at GCRO council meetings under that misnomer 'any other business'. The GCRO had originally arisen from the wreckage of the House of Lords Select Committee Report on the Osteopaths Bill (1935). Unconsciously, the council reflected its members' own defensiveness. They appeared to excuse themselves for existing as osteopaths and were frightened and perhaps hurt by the previous debacle in 1935 and worried about the repercussions should Fielding fail in his endeavour.

The first step required was seeking allies outside the GCRO council, beyond those already well trusted within the inner circle of family and ESO colleagues. To start with Fielding was introduced to Nigel Clarke who had been involved in Conservative Central Office and had intimate knowledge of how to organise political campaigns. He regarded Private Members' bills as inadequate vehicles with which to promote legislation. The Ministry of Health would have to back any successful statutory regulation and attempts had to be made to gain its support. It was also important to address and rebut medical opposition to such legal proposals and anticipate any arguments.[4] One plan of action was to make some sort of personal acknowledgement to those who were indifferent or even hostile. Clarke suggested that Fielding's message needed to be succinct, clear and light-hearted but also couched in humour and goodwill.

Despite all of these efforts, in May 1986 the BMA report on alternative therapies including osteopathy was at best indifferent to its value, and at worse, highly negative. Conversely, the national press and a number of politicians were critical of the BMA report's conclusions and their attitude towards osteopathy in general. It was Clarke who orchestrated a strategy for the next step, financed by the OGF. Harold Klug and Robert Lever, co-OGF colleagues, who had helped before, devoted considerable support to this mission too.[5]

In the early 1980s, the OGF had commissioned a survey from Medicare to ascertain basic facts such as exactly what osteopaths did in practice. From this enquiry certain points became clear, for example, training covered a wide spectrum: including diplomas awarded after two weekends of study; bona fide extended pathway courses without clinical provision; full-time degree courses; and even postgraduate courses for medical students. The findings gave Fielding and Clarke ammunition for politicians to further the urgency for state regulation. Osteopaths had to demonstrate credible training standards and upgrade those schools needing to improve and maintain these standards.

In 1986, Fielding with Tony Durant's help, GCRO cooperation and Clarke's manoeuvres, decided to fly a kite in the form of an idea doomed to fail, as an effective way of measuring parliamentary support for statutory regulation. Firstly, he and Clarke cobbled together an eight page dossier based on the *Optician's Bill*, which he dispatched to a number of registered osteopaths in different constituencies so that they could find out whether their MPs would support a similar bill for osteopaths. Many phone calls were required to motivate at the grassroots level but they responded well. Feedback showed that the majority of MPs were willing to back such a proposal. Under a ten minute bill, Roy Galley MP introduced a motion to statutorily regulate osteopaths. As expected it failed to gain any motivation in the Commons, but it did cause quite a stir among those osteopaths outside the GCRO.

There was considerable outcry and flak from some practitioners who genuinely believed that their livelihoods might be wrested from them. Many waged bitter vitriol; Clarke and Fielding's efforts had led to personal denigration. Future attempts to achieve state regulation had to include the support of all osteopaths, allaying the mistrust and venom some felt for the GCRO. Allies began to be sought within this disgruntled group and to a vision extended beyond a GCRO-inspired registration body. In fact, the GCRO did appear to be too parochial to use as a vehicle for transferring regulatory powers. Clarke and Fielding began to think beyond its perimeters. Discussions became a relentless game that had to be played with the civil servant given the task of negotiating. Fruitless days were spent traipsing the well-worn routes of unfeasible propositions like the *Professions Supplementary to Medicine Act*, which was a method the establishment used to block progress. No alternative group had been state regulated since homeopathic physicians under the *Medical Act* of 1858.

Whilst the civil servant was immovable, his replacement, Robyn Balderstone, offered a sea change. Fielding and Clarke found her very enthusiastic, friendly, and willing to advance the process forward. She arranged an appointment with Lord Skelmersdale, Secretary of State for Health. Skelmersdale, a hereditary peer and a true blue aristocrat with a very dry sense of humour, stipulated that the cause required clear-cut aims. The talks concluded with four tenets: the medical profession would have to support the application; there had to be a consensus among the whole osteopathic profession, even those who vehemently opposed the GCRO; education standards must be upgraded and upheld; and ethical criteria approved. Everything would be bound around these principles. This connection introduced Clarke and Fielding to the sympathetic ear of Lord Kindersley, who managed to obtain a debate in the House of Lords on the subject. The Lords Baldwin, Cullen of Ashbourne, and Colwyn, friends of osteopathy, were given folders written by Fielding, Clarke and Balderstone, to help them during the deliberations. At last, things were progressing and it was Kindersley who would advance the cause now even further.[6]

A close friend of the Prince of Wales, Kindersley advised Fielding and Clarke that the Prince's involvement might speed up the whole process. A proposal was devised. The Prince would invite the Health Minister, the Right Honourable Tony Newton MP, Sir Raymond Hoffenberg, President of the Royal Physicians, Ian Todd, President of the Royal College of Surgeons, Lord Walton, President of the General Medical Council, President of the British Medical Association, Colin Dove, Kindersley, Fielding and some civil servants, to Kensington Palace for a private lunch.

Until the main course had been eaten, conversation of a general nature flowed around the table. The Prince of Wales then announced the lunch's main purpose and proposed discourse on statutory regulation of osteopaths. He asked Fielding to explain the reasons behind implementing such a programme. Fielding outlined the four bedrocks: professional unity; upgraded osteopathic education to a uniform standard; upheld professional ethics; and approval and support of the medical profession. The Prince replied that this seemed a splendid idea and he went round the table to his medical guests asking them to discuss the matter with Fielding at future meetings. They all acceded to his request; he finished by asking Newton if the government could expedite its recommendation. Newton equivocated over its procedure through Parliament, claiming it would not be in the interest of the government to interfere. Finally, the Prince thanked everyone for attending and explained that he would be in regular contact with Fielding to hear how all the talks were progressing.

This lunch was the icebreaker, not only opening a long-awaited dialogue with the main medical institutions, but also taking Clarke and Fielding away from GCRO self-interest towards other allies (including the Prince of Wales), and tackling the whole profession's welfare. It was Tony Newton, a thoughtful man of deep integrity, who accompanied by Fielding spoke at the convention of one osteopathic group outside the GCRO. He outlined Skelmersdale's four tenets for statutory regulation, which would form the basis of advancing the profession. He further proposed with Skelmersdale's help that all osteopathic schools and colleges should be independently inspected. Clarke and Fielding realised nothing could be attained without support from the entire body of osteopaths *and* medical endorsement. In this way the fears of both groups could be allayed whilst at the same time the statutory proposals could be fostered.

The next question was how to gain support from a diverse spectrum of educational establishments. Many of the schools were mistrustful of the proposed statutory regulation and the role of the GCRO council in its preparation. The Osteopathic Genesis Foundation (OGF) was prepared to fund an independent report on all of the schools under the British Accreditation Council (BAC) auspices accompanied by Dr Dudley Tee and Professor Irwin Korr. Constant reassurance was needed to placate almost pathological suspicion, bordering on hatred in a few. Diplomacy was used to encourage those schools that approved upgraded standards to seek assistance, thereby leading to credible, acceptable courses.

Meanwhile, Jane Langer of the College of Osteopaths (COET) played the definitive role in placating fears, understanding that each osteopathic institution had to make substantial concessions if osteopathic unity was to metamorphose from a distant dream into a practical reality. It was at a meeting of the Committee of Complementary and Alternative Medicine that Langer was told the vacant seat next to her was taken by Fielding of the dreaded GCRO. During an interval for refreshments she sought him out, hoping to destroy any ideas that she and her

COET colleagues were against professional unity. It was a wish she shared with her father who had been a pioneer at the BSO in his day. Fielding, in ebullient style, flung his arms around her, saying, "I've met someone who thinks like me, will you work with me?" Here was a person who could disarm groups deeply suspicious of what they saw as the GCRO taking over the profession and swallowing up smaller associations.[7] Fielding and Clarke recognised that Langer had the resolve to bring about momentous shifts within the profession. They accepted that support for statutory regulation was contained within two pillars: unification of the whole osteopathic profession; and medical bodies' approval.

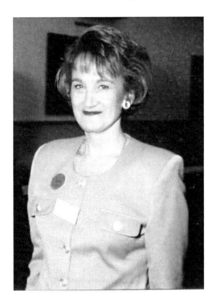

Fig. 26: Jane Langer

Fielding's initial meeting with medical groups was held at the Royal College of Physicians and was accompanied by Sir Raymond Hoffenberg. Clarke had taught Fielding that without any personal connection, conversations of this nature could be stilted and awkward. Hoffenberg was a South African who had known Fielding's grandfather during his days in that country and this link made conversation easier. Hoffenberg proceeded to assist him and over three meetings he was able to gain some acknowledgement, not only with the Royal College of Physicians but also its umbrella organisation, the Royal Faculties. The Royal College of Surgeons proved somewhat harder to budge but Fielding overcame some of the difficulty by reminding Ian Todd that Fielding's own wife had been a valuable member of

Todd's surgical team. Once on board, Todd arranged a lunch with his orthopaedic colleagues who were opposed to such a bill. Fortunately it appears that the orthopods had reluctantly agreed to back their other colleagues.

Fielding's next step was to negotiate with Lord Walton and Professor Crisp, Director of Education, at the GMC Headquarters. Walton, an outstanding neurologist, proposed various clinical scenarios presenting in practice and grilled him intently on neurology. The viva continued until Walton and Crisp appeared satisfied that Fielding seemingly knew his subject, the limitations of practice, clinical boundaries, specific red flags and when to refer patients to general practitioners. Walton was an astute politician, appearing to show support for the proposition while perhaps just being differential.[8] He did warn Fielding that the BMA were formidable opponents to the notion of statutory regulation of osteopaths.

In 1987, the BMA published a report on osteopathy describing it in a far from positive light. Its higher echelons were very dismissive of the profession. On various meetings with their president, Fielding was able to allay fears that osteopaths wished to take over aspects of their work. He reiterated the fact that the public should expect well-trained practitioners with considerable ethical standards. Slowly, BMA opinion shifted towards support. Finally their president stated that the Association had no right in standing in their way. Later, Tara Lamont redrafted the original BMA report, highlighting some support for osteopathy.[9] Once Fielding had informed the Prince of Wales that progress had was being made with medical institutions, HRH as President of the King's Fund approached it with a view to setting up a working party to review statutory regulation.[10]

The King's Fund working party on Statutory Regulation of Osteopaths was formed in 1989 under the chairmanship of Sir Thomas Bingham, a brilliant judge who was later to become Lord Chief Justice. He was an intellectual with a capacity to grasp minutiae quickly and did allow any one person to dominate proceedings. Fielding advised the King's Fund to appoint Langer to represent groups outside the GCRO and also Dr John Armitstead, a consultant physician and osteopath. Together with Fielding they formed a triumvirate representing osteopathic interests. The medical side was represented by the familiar faces of Sir John Walton (GMC president) and Ian Todd (President of the Royal College of Surgeons). They were joined by Dr David Shaw (Newcastle University Medical School), an expert on healthcare education. Annabel Ford, a journalist specialising in health, plus two observers completed the working party. Its secretary was Lord Illingworth. The osteopathic trio was initially a bit apprehensive but Bingham made certain that they had an equal chance to voice their views and soon these evening meetings were held in a convivial atmosphere.[11]

In total there were seventeen meetings, each lasting about an hour. It was made implicit that these people had read the relevant papers before each assembly. During one of these sessions non-GCRO osteopathic associations, mistrustful of the working party's considerations, were invited to meet its committee members. Within a short time Bingham had disarmed their hostilities and allayed their fears in the same manner that he had used with the medical representatives in earlier sessions. Possibly one of the greatest judges of the last century, the profession owes Bingham much in driving his working party forward with drafting the bill. It was good fortune too that all the members were of a high calibre and the stimulating sittings gathered impetus towards legislation.

On 1st July 1993, almost a century after JM Littlejohn gave his first talks about osteopathy on British soil, the *Osteopaths Act* received Royal Assent. The Act led to the establishment of the General Osteopathic Council (GOsC), which took over the GCRO's responsibility. The first Statutory Register of Osteopaths was produced in 2000. At last the profession had a united front supported by the legislation that so many had campaigned for.

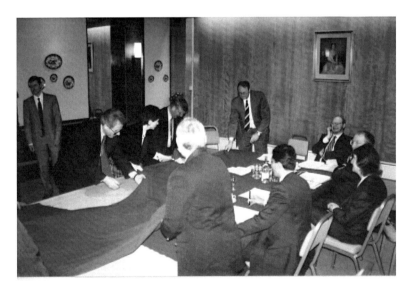

Fig. 27: First meeting of the GOsC

Analysis

The first step in the direction towards achieving state legislation was made by the appointment of Peter Blaker as GCRO secretary. He oversaw the transition of the largest voluntary registered group of osteopaths into a professional, reasonably organised, ethically aware institution. It was clearly important to demonstrate to others that the profession could make such a change. For that, osteopaths owe Blaker a considerable amount of gratitude. On completion, Blaker's position and that of the GCRO became superfluous. Both had fulfilled their tasks and their roles were no longer relevant to the process of statutory regulation.

A much bigger concept now embraced the whole osteopathic profession. In 1986, several important factors coalesced. The BMA report on alternative medicine reflected an official medical view of osteopathy in negative terms although subsequently some of the national press and politicians critically rounded on the report. Meanwhile, the OGF continued to fund various projects, assisting Fielding's parliamentary activities. Nigel Clarke began to help him with strategic aims. A Private Members' Bill had no success but Ministry of Health endorsement was essential if statutory regulation was to be achieved. The reasons why there was some medical opposition to regulation were considered carefully and osteopathic rebuttals of them given.

Clarke provided pragmatic advice while Lever and Klug gave Fielding much needed osteopathic counsel. It was a change of civil servant that opened the door to Lord Skelmersdale, Minister of State, Health and later, Tony Newton, Secretary of State, Ministry of Health. Four indisputable precepts were outlined. At the pivotal lunch arranged by the Prince of Wales key figures were introduced. Behind the scenes, Clarke assisted Fielding with discussions about strategy and helped to familiarise him with their medical doubts and fears. Although Fielding could have amicable meetings with them, this does not mean that favourable views continued within the confines of their specific institutions.

The Prince of Wales suggested a King's Fund working party should be setup under the chairmanship of Sir Thomas Bingham. Both Newton and Bingham played essential parts in its successful outcome. Fielding was also ably assisted by Jane Langer, who spent interminable evenings on the phone reassuring non-GCRO osteopaths of progress and was responsible, ultimately, for their continued support. Without her contribution all other efforts were doomed to fail. Equally important was John Armitstead, consultant physician and osteopath, seen as the acceptable osteopathic face of reason and moderation. He performed a similar role to that taken on by Kelman MacDonald half a century earlier during the ill-fated House of

Lords Select Committee. Armitstead's presence must have had quite an effect on Lord Walton and Ian Todd, both consummate politicians. The working party was able to plan a blueprint for statutory regulation for osteopaths to proceed through Parliament towards Royal Assent.

There were a number of pivotal moments within the process but two key ones were the Prince of Wales's lunch and Bingham's chairmanship of the working party. Osteopathic history also benefits from the work of many key figures during this period of its evolution. Robyn Balderstone, Lord Skelmersdale and Tony Newton all shared special civil servant and governmental roles, supporting statutory regulation. Peter Blaker under the GCRO chairmanship of Barry Lambert transformed the voluntary Register into a professional outfit. In the background, Robert Lever and Harold Klug gave endless time and backing. Nigel Clarke became indispensable during the procedure. Jane Langer and John Armitstead were invaluable colleagues as Simon Fielding enacted his essential part as conduit. Whether statutory regulation has fulfilled all our aspirations is another thing, but for their efforts, we owe these people much.

References

1. Blaker Peter, NOA DVD Interview. 2008.
2. Ibid.
3. Ibid.
4. Clarke, Nigel, NOA DVD Interview. 2008.
5. Fielding, Simon, NOA DVD Volume 1 Statutory Regulation of Osteopaths Interview. 2009.
6. Ibid.
7. Langer, Jane, NOA DVD Interview. 2008.
8. Pembury, Dr. Susan, Personal Interview. 2011.
9. Fielding.
10. Armitstead, John, NOA DVD Interview. 2008.
11. Langer.

Chapter 10

Cranial Osteopathy in Britain

Précis

One of the most intriguing aspects of osteopathic history involves the origin and growth of cranial osteopathy. Its probable American roots emerged from phrenology in the 1830s and magnetic healing a decade later. These two groups intertwined briefly to form phreno-magnetism, which appears to be a precursor of cranial osteopathy. One of the early pioneers of cranial osteopathy, William Garner Sutherland, hypothesised that various dysfunctions were caused by the minute displacement of cranial bones. A small cohort of dedicated practitioners under the Cranial Academy (CA) and the Sutherland Cranial Teaching Foundation (SCTF) proselytised Sutherland's discrete concept.

In the 1950s, Eddie Gilhooley and others pioneered its practice in the UK. Links were made with the SCTF, which flourished for some time. Cranial osteopathy grew in popularity and demand in Britain, becoming an integral part of undergraduate training. At a time when statutory regulation in the UK hinged on the approval of all osteopaths, a series of misunderstandings arose between the American Osteopathic Association authorities and UK course directors over non-registered osteopaths attending these SCTF sponsored courses. Although cranial osteopathy developed on the margins of the profession, its value has since been realised in mainstream practice.

Historical Examination

In order to consider the origins of cranial osteopathy it is necessary to go back a long way to the early part of the nineteenth century when phrenology first appeared in the USA, followed a decade later by mesmerism. Phrenology hypothesised that 'lumps and bumps' on the cranial bones caused pressure on identifiable aspects of the brain, which phrenologists surmised as being centres influencing the very nature of the individual. It was thought that their presence caused various forms of dysfunction. Many were perplexed by its premise that sociological dysfunction could be caused by lumps and bumps to the cranium and was not perpetrated by the devil incarnate. Critics following this train of thought concluded that it represented blasphemy at its most profound and implied that the Divine did not exist in the way that had been taught and worshipped. These contentious views were reclaimed by mesmerism, which appeared to come to the salvation of phrenology by suggesting that universal energy entered the skull and flowed throughout the body to somehow nullify the negative effects of these cranial defects. Mesmerism stated that a lack of universal energy caused dysfunction in the soul, mind and body of an individual. They called this flow magnetism, electricity, universal energy, god flow, spiritual energy, and Holy Spirit.

We know that for some time AT Still advertised himself as a "magnetic healer". He also helped his father to care for his Methodist Circuit. The mission was located at a crossing of the Missouri River, a point passed by thousands of settlers on their way west. In 1858 Still was involved in a disruption Missouri Compromise, an edict to balance the interests of slave states against 'free' States. This breach saw pro-slavery and abolitionists' irregular forces participating in guerrilla warfare and skirmishes over proclaimed indigenous native territory to form the new state of Kansas. The campaign of land appropriation became known as "Bleeding Kansas", a forerunner of Union versus Confederacy and later its resultant American Civil War. Abolitionist recruits from New England and other east coast states brought new ideas of healing which influenced Still and his compatriots on the Unionist side. Magnetic healing had emanated from European roots in Austria and France and gained some success on the east coast. It developed two fold, as medical hypnosis and as a public spectacle in the form of rudimentary psychology. In a sense it was a 'mother' therapy, spawning religious groups, psychotherapeutic movements and manipulative therapies.

It was Phineas Parkhurst Quimby (1802–66) who fine-tuned magnetic healing into a psychological therapy to treat depressed people. He derived his successes from building a rapport between patient and therapist. Emerging from this relationship, healing took place in a safe, secure atmosphere. Quimby explained about health and disease to the patient in a matter-of-fact way.[1] In doing so he stumbled upon ways not only to enhance the placebo effect, but also an unexpected yet crucial link between physical and psychological dysfunction. Magnetic healers perceived recovery as an adjustment within a person's metaphysical dimension rather than within their physical or psychological nature.[2] Nonetheless, they were superficially aware of the complex relationship between beliefs, emotions and the behaviour of their patients.[3] They described conditions in terms of energy or 'bodily fluid' blockages, an interesting view that Still would tweak, taking it from a quasi-religious crusade to the secular world, emphasising physical adjustment and spinal displacement in restoring general health.[4]

It can be postulated there was a substantial psychological element to osteopathy which has been neglected by others. Perhaps Still did not envisage physical and

psychological disorders being separate but saw their systems as interacting together. He just could not explain this phenomenon satisfactorily and instead he
described things in language difficult to construe. Meanwhile, on Quimby's death
in 1866, his followers continued to proselytise his therapy. Mary Baker Eddy wrote
a poetic eulogy but very gradually distanced herself from Quimby to found her
Christian Science movement.[5] Others such as Warren Felt Evans set up metaphysical clubs that were scattered around various states including Kansas. It is possible
that Still was influenced by such institutions.

By 1874 Still was practising as a magnetic healer, much to the dismay of his family
and local Methodist church in Baldwin. He decided to travel to nearby Kirksville
where the community was more tolerant and he rented rooms for practice. Still
practised exclusively as a magnetic healer until the late 1870s. His approach
depended on Quimby's hypothesis that unless patients trusted a practitioner they
could not regain health. Although Still's practice eventually declined, magnetic
healing gave him the necessary clinical strategies not only to enhance the placebo
effect but also some chance of improving chronic physical conditions. Moreover,
once he had added bonesetting to his skill set he could treat long-standing
psychosomatic and related illness in a psychological and physical way while
offering a physical explanation. Consequently, throughout the 1880s he advertised
himself as a "lightning bonesetter".[6]

William Garner Sutherland was interested in cranial bones and the complexity of
their interrelated sutures. He proposed that cranial bones could be somehow in
lesion by being marginally out of place, and that in some specific cranial locality its
dynamic subtle motion may be impaired causing certain dysfunction. Sutherland
called this study cranial osteopathy.

By 1945, phrenology had been extinguished as an alternative medical therapy.
However, its demise coincided with a gradual increase of interest in cranial
osteopathy in the US and latterly in the UK. In Britain, Edward Gilhooley, an
Aberdonian osteopath, maintained a considerable long-term interest and correspondence with Sutherland and his Cranial Academy of Osteopathy throughout
the 1950s until his death at the end of decade.[7] Gilhooley attended at least one
cranial convention in America. At the same time we also have information that
Robert Lowe, a well-known Lancashire osteopath, had studied Sutherland's papers
and literally learnt its craft from the notes.[8]

Eventually it was Denis Brookes, a great friend of Eddie Gilhooley, who proselytised cranial osteopathy in the UK and Continental Europe. He emerged as a
decisive influence during the 1960s and Gilhooley might well have played an

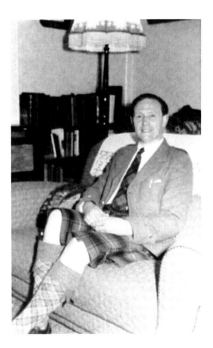

Fig. 28: Eddie Gilhooley

important part in Brookes' training. Among these early UK exponents was Emilie Jackson, a Kirksville graduate whose family was steeped in traditional osteopathy. At this time the American Osteopathy Association's (AOA) Cranial Academy (CA) had begun to send out a few practitioners including Harold Magoun and Viola Frymann to London and Paris in the 1960s. In France, Jacques Duval, a 1963 BSO graduate and gold medallist, became a regular member of these courses in Britain and America too. He played a crucial role in constructing a cordial relationship between American osteopathic physicians and European osteopathy. In the late 1960s the triumvirate of Denis Brookes, 'Sam' Grierson Currie and John Dixon, criticised the British School of Osteopathy (BSO) board for not broadening the scope of the curriculum to include cranial osteopathy.

Meanwhile there was a growing public interest in alternative medicine: chiropractic; osteopathy; homeopathy; acupuncture; psychoanalysis; meditation and yoga. By now, due to the rise in vaccinations, the impact of certain illnesses on children had declined markedly. But to some extent scientific advancements were at the expense of a loss of personal touch from medical staff. In earlier practise, human interaction was really the only thing available to offer. By contrast, alternative therapists appeared to prescribe these sometimes missing particular, individual touches as well as seeming to refer to some higher quality of life.

Even if this appeared to be a golden age of alternative medicine with no mandatory need to adopt evidence-based approval, some osteopaths were in fact questioning the relevance of the biophysical model initiated by the BSO two decades before. Its construct was perhaps too narrowly defined and rather two-dimensional in concept. Yet Audrey Smith of the BSO had developed osteopathic diagnosis away from the "bony lesion" to include a pathological sieve. She designed a four-year curriculum to acknowledge the complexity of her biopathophysical concept. Its critics appeared to come from two ends of the osteopathic spectrum. Some biomechanics thought there were additional components, psychosocial and stress-related factors.[9] More artistically inclined osteopaths were ready to extend their training to include cranial and, perhaps, transfer their practice to one not dominated by 'whack, crack and thwack' thrust techniques. There seemed to be a yearning to be freed from the musculoskeletal ghetto, and to step towards cranial osteopathy and other specialisms including visceral treatment. At this point a few cranial practitioners were willing to spread Sutherland's message.

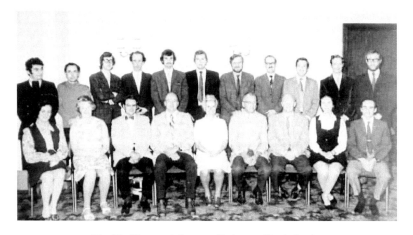

Fig. 29: First cranial course, Ecclestone Hotel, London

In 1972, Grierson Currie arranged a cranial course at the Ecclestone Hotel, London. Jacques Duval and Martin Pascoe assisted him and 14 further BSO graduates attended including a sceptical Colin Dove, then BSO principal.[10] Four American cranial stalwarts, Harold Magoun, Tom Scholey, John Harakal and Viola Frymann, were principle lecturers.[11] Dove had been persuaded to attend by the BSO board of directors who sought to pacity Currie et al who continued to exhort its inclusion in the BSO curriculum. Meanwhile, Magoun propounded Sutherland's somewhat outmoded 'bony lesion' notion, which seemed to dismay Dove and others. The BSO hypothesis of a pathophysiological dysfunction model appeared streets ahead.

Sutherland's hypothesis was undergoing some change in the American Academy of Osteopathy too. An essential one was the establishment of a cranial rhythm and its arrythmical dysfunction. Novitiates were expected to feel this subtle expansion and contraction of the skull. Many felt they could ascertain cranial movement and developed practices on such claims. Others postulated that it was cerebrospinal fluid motion which could be perceptively felt along its route. Many supporters nowadays view cranial osteopathy as a subtle, variable form of communication between two persons, the practitioner and client. The practitioner uses his own stillness as a neutral force, transferring this tranquillity via a possible trance-like state dynamically to the client. It is postulated that this allows the client to benefit from an opening-up experience, a broadening of their cognitive scope whilst the practitioner experientially builds up a database of subtle palpation: hard, tight, tight, loose, boggy appreciation of tissue.[12] At the heart of cranial osteopathy's development has been the AOA's Cranial Academy (CA) and the Sutherland Cranial Teaching Foundation (SCTF).

In 1973, Dove wrote to Don Woods, a member of the AOA House of Delegates asking him to look into AOA plans to celebrate the centenary of Still's "unfurling of the banner of osteopathy in 1874". His letter also included comments on the previous year's course aftermath. He had discovered he could not find time to practise its methods and in any case believed it was unlikely to progress in Britain. In his reply, Woods stated they had made no plans to celebrate osteopathy's centenary but he did invite Dove to attend the CA and AOA meetings in Colorado Springs officially as a BSO faculty member.[13] Furthermore, the SCTF had awarded him a scholarship to cover his costs. It was the first time the AOA had accorded any official response to the BSO or its representative since 1925, although official invitations had been made in the past to members of the British Osteopathic Association (BOA), graduates of AOA affiliated colleges and those with medical degrees. BSO directors were reluctant to support cranial osteopathy but felt it was politically expedient to strengthen their rather tenuous links with American counterparts. They gave Dove financial help and official approval to attend the cranial course at the Eisenhower Memorial Hospital in Colorado Springs.[14]

At this AOA conference Dove received much support from the indefatigable Jacques Duval. Both could not sympathise with the rationale taught, finding too much emphasis on bony lesion ethos, inexplicable axes of motion, rigid osteological concepts rather than living tissue elasticity and incomprehensible prescriptive treatment of specific osteopathic techniques applied to clinical syndromes. The CA conference followed where fortunately the great Rollin Becker filled in for the absent Phil Greenman. He outlined in his usual charismatic way ideas of dysfunctional causation affecting the whole body instead of the rigid bony lesion concept. Becker could be gruff and monosyllabic in private but his lively public oratory and individual tutoring methods found resonance with Duval and Dove. They enrolled for the next CA convention the following year in Louisville, Kentucky, together with Martin Pascoe. This time Dove was invited to give a paper. Becker was present as a faculty member and executive director of the SCTF. This conference introduced the European trio to Ann Wales, a former student of Sutherland, and also the cranial maestros Bob Fulford and Herb Miller. The CA meeting that followed laid the foundations of a formal relationship between the American SCTF and the BSO postgraduate department. Presiding over all this must have been the ghost of JM Littlejohn with his "vibratility caused by a vital force" concept, not too dissimilar from Becker's total "body phenomenon".[15]

The SCTF committed to providing lecturers for a postgraduate course organised under the auspices of the BSO just for medical and dental practitioners. General Council and Registered Osteopaths (GCRO) were also permitted to attend. In private, Becker as SCTF executive had enormous trust in Dove to run the UK side of operations without any US interference. Unfortunately, Becker had no authorisation to do such a thing. He did bequeath Dove personal control of the BSO/GCRO postgraduate intake. Although the BSO board were reluctant, they eventually subscribed to such a quest.

During that year the BSO board laid down two provisos before sanctioning the new course: Colin Dove must retain overall control as course director; and it was to be designated postgraduate study only. There followed a series of annual SCTF/BSO postgraduate cranial courses attended by Dove, Viola Frymann and Tom Scholey in 1974, Rollin Becker and John Harakal in 1975 and Edna Lay in 1976. The following year Dove retired as BSO principal and the reluctant BSO directors continued to be resolute, if not more unyielding about including cranial osteopathy in the BSO curriculum. Be that as it may, the new BSO principal asked Dove to become the director of a newly established department of Postgraduate Studies where the SCTF/BSO annual course would remain centre stage. Many of the American cranial doyens lectured at these sessions: Ann Wales; Alan and Rollin Becker; John Harakal; Herb and Ed Miller; and Jim Jealous. Students also benefitted from the irresistible osteopathic interpretation of Bob Fulford.[16] The developing dialogue between American osteopathic physicians and British osteopaths had been built on strong personal bonds between Dove and Rollin Becker initially and later, John Harakal. What was assumed to be verbal agreements between them was apparently not conveyed to the SCTF board. However, Jealous has stated these conversations were communicated to them but they were never ratified.[17]

In 1985 while the SCTF/BSO courses were successful and fully booked, Sutherland's ideas were being spread throughout osteopathic groups in Europe and the Antipodes. Dove had been appointed associate SCTF board member, evidence of his valuable work, integrity and professionalism. It was not his only contribution. For many years he had maintained a correspondence with Tom Dummer. Dove sympathised with him about the general osteopathic disunity existing amidst a myriad of small splintered groups. One of the ways that some dialogue could be addressed was through avant-garde groups such as cranial. Sometime in the early 1980s Dove spoke to Becker about allowing the Society of Osteopaths (SO) and graduates of the European School of Osteopathy (ESO) onto the SCTF/BSO courses. Becker acceded to Dove's knowledge and agreed that they should attend. Dove pointed out to Becker that they would gain GCRO membership in the near future. Similarly, Dove worked with Michael van Straten to persuade John Harakal, SCTF president, to agree to British College of Naturopathy and Osteopathy (BCNO) graduates taking the course despite their GCRO ineligibility. Harakal approved of this verbally too. There were risks attached to these premature arrangements but Dove, from his side, was proven correct. Clearly, SCTF board arrangements were only loosely communicated during these times and no one criticised Dove's commitment, worth and industry during these heady, booming days. Things started to fragment at the very time that this small but contentious cranial group appeared to flourish.

Meanwhile, John Harakal at the end of 1984 had written to Dove to clear up a discrepancy occurring in Belgium.[18] Some BCNO graduates had applied to enter the Brussels SCTF course but it was Harakal's notion that only Maidstone (ESO) and BSO groups were allowed to join the SCTF courses. Dove notes in his reply:

"Where we have taken some licence, and not without consultation, although neither Rollin (Becker) nor I seem to have put it on paper, was in accepting Society (SO) members and later BNOA (British Naturopathic and Osteopathic Association) members in advance of their admission as MROs (GCRO members). However to have treated the BNOA less fairly and to deny them now (unless the GCRO refuses them which is unlikely) would have been a damaging step."[19]

There is enough evidence from GCRO minutes too that matters were progressing towards increasing professional unity but at a very slow rate with some intermittent blips. It is surprising that their long-time dutiful registrar, Richard Miller, should be one of those reluctant to push things forward when he himself had joined the GCRO as an article eleven entrant (i.e. one who has not been trained at an accredited school), a clause that was closed shortly after his entry. Moreover, things had developed within the AOA hierarchy following the Brussels debacle. Harakal's subsequent correspondence contains two important events which took place from the SCTF Board. Firstly, Dove was elected to join the SCTF as an associate director and, secondly, a month later in September 1985, Harakal informed him of details from the American Academy of Osteopathy and AOA who were looking "to limit educational opportunities for all osteopaths/osteopathic physicians not holding American DO degrees".[20] It is likely that the latter outcome was brought about by the Brussels furore. In reply, Dove pronounced:

"The BSO is eternally grateful to the SCTF for their great help in fostering this work. In this regard the 1985 AOA decision not to allow its members to teach osteopaths unless they are destined for full licensure (US DO degree), is shutting the stable door after the horse has bolted. It is a sad decision for political reasons by those (as political decisions usually are) who are not in complete possession of all of the facts…(UK Osteopathy) managed to get established, grew and developed over 70 years without the AOA and as we are now growing at a faster pace than ever before (the profession will double its size between 1985 and 1990), we can manage quite easily without the AOA for the next 70!"[21]

In some respects the success of the BSO postgraduate-centred courses had progressed cranial training to a position whereby many of the early UK postgraduate students had rather outgrown their American teachers. In fact, later courses only featured one American SCTF speaker. Clearly, in one sense their UK counterparts could manage quite effectively without this existing umbilical relationship. From Dove's point of view it was an honour to receive an SCTF associate directorship, but at the same time he knew that very few UK individuals could attend board meetings in the USA on a regular basis, hence it was an honour but one devoid of any practical application. His transatlantic endeavours were reliant on fragile, rather tenuous 'nod and wink' agreements with Becker and Harakal. It must have seemed ironic, perhaps even farcical to him that he was grappling with a GCRO going through the slow transformation of opening up its membership to other accredited schools and their alumni associations. Furthermore, he was

115

attempting to facilitate broader postgraduate attendance on a SCTF-sponsored BSO cranial course by including worthy ESO and BCNO graduates, not as yet eligible for GCRO inclusion.

At the same time Dove had to understand perplexing dealings with the Applied Academy of Osteopathy (AAO) and the American Osteopathic Association (AOA) and their directives to exclude all bar US-trained DOs on their courses. Meanwhile, US SCTF individual members were at liberty to lecture, tutor and support groups not AOA affiliated and they had by now not only viewed their British counterparts as colleagues but also many had made deep friendships.[22] John Upledger, a charismatic and influential American DO, went further and organised training courses in his institute outside the osteopathic domain. The American SCTF continued to sponsor postgraduate courses beyond the USA for doctors, dentists and equivalent GCRO osteopaths. Yet in the US these courses were exclusively for US DOs only. It was all very confusing. To overcome such hurdles study groups took to bypassing any AAO/AOA official activities. A congenial transatlantic dialogue continued to take place without retribution despite unofficial recognition of these contacts. By the end of 1987, Colin Dove "delegated the task of course director to Nick Woodhead, with John Harakal's approval".[23]

Dove continued to be overall BSO Director of Postgraduate Studies and approved associate SCTF director/board member. It has to be reiterated that the early Anglo-American cranial links forged with Dove and Becker had been based on mutual trust. Such a set-up continued with John Harakal after Becker's serious stroke. He too formed a good, mutually trusting relationship with Dove until he also succumbed to illness. The young practitioner Michael Burruano had only recently joined the SCTF board, but he was catapulted prematurely into the presidency. Burruano was from a different generation, very respectful of his elders on the board but, naturally more in tune with his own generation.[24] The gentleman's handshake-like relationship that had existed between Dove, Becker and Harakal did not continue in the same way with Burruano, although this was through the fault of no one. Dove's involvement in allowing non-GCRO osteopaths onto courses had led a number of SCTF board members to remain suspicious of his motives. Becker and Harakal had acceded to this and Jealous confirmed that the subject had been mentioned at official board meetings but was never ratified. To these members it was not a small matter but one that the AAO/AOA had deliberated about although they did finally decide to refuse non-US-trained DOs further access to courses on American soil. The problem arose again in the early 1990s.

By July 1990 the BSO was crippled by enormous debts. Clive Standen, BSO principal, decided to close the Postgraduate Studies department even though it had made some profit. Dove no longer had a job but he resigned anyway as its director, yet SCTF support for him continued as an associate director and board member. Many of the BSO cranial postgraduate faculty had been subsumed into teaching cranial training at undergraduate level at the school under the direction of Martin Pascoe. In addition, Dove's attendance at the infrequently held SCTF board meeting was impractical, making his role of associate board member more honorary than purposeful. Besides, UK osteopathy was proceeding towards statutory regulation and ultimately towards a unified profession. Unfortunately, Dove's health deteriorated rapidly, culminating in major heart surgery. He had been present at the forefront of cranial osteopathy for two decades, initially as a healthy sceptic and then acknowledging Rollin Becker's outstanding contribution to furthering Sutherland's premise. He became convinced of a potential in the cranial hypothesis, organised postgraduate courses and cemented cordial transatlantic relations. Unfortunately, the profession has relied on too few individuals such as Colin Dove to manage its affairs. Even with a BSO ethos to work in teams rather than at the behest of gurus, it was extremely difficult for groups to function democratically, appearing to accept the toil of specific persons.

Many osteopaths had joined the profession as resolute individualists who were prepared to speak their own version or that held by their pundit, but were unable to listen, discuss and debate without veering from the point at issue or descending into personal invective. This theme of misunderstanding, misinterpretation and personal diatribe ran through the autistic annals of osteopathy. The GCRO was an attempt to address these failings but it hardly offered a blueprint of tolerance for others to adopt. No one in the Sutherland Cranial Course (SCC) that emerged from British SCTF faculty teachers had any cohesive notion about how to run things, just managing instead to provide an agreed ethos and promote Sutherland's work. A steering committee was formed of Sue Turner, Nick Handoll, Caroline Penn, Martin Pascoe, Joyce Vetterlein and Nick Woodhead, who had been director of the BSO postgraduate course for the past four years. There was no reason to believe that the new committee would not actually benefit UK cranial osteopathy. Meanwhile, the BSO's postgraduate department was closed due to financial constraints caused by plummeting BSO funds. Clive Standen, BSO principal, felt that the high level courses could continue under a new arrangement. They were financially successful and did make a significant financial contribution to BSO's meagre resources. The unofficial links with American SCTF members continued to flourish without referring back to the SCTF board. Students kept to an SCTF syllabus and transatlantic goodwill prospered. While Dove rehabilitated from surgery, the steering committee met three or four times.

Much of the transatlantic rapprochement had been conducted by a few people. The steering committee was aware their constitution needed to reflect a more democratic and clearer ethos. Yet whilst the committee felt grateful for Dove's efforts, there needed to be a greater distribution of effort and a wider dissemination of agreed notions among a larger number of faculty members. Michael Burruano was fully aware of this situation too.

While all acceded to this, the central issue that could not be discounted even with a majority consensus was the hoary chestnut of allowing non-GCRO members onto the courses. It became a key topic for discussion.[25] Many of the BSO postgraduate course tutors were teaching on the BSO student course run by Martin Pascoe, ably assisted by Nick Woodhead. They were fully aware of the Brussels course misgivings within the US SCTF board and beyond within the AAO and AOA. Any group blocking the attendance of non-GCRO members in Britain would always get a sympathetic hearing in the USA. Pascoe at first and then later Woodhead as well felt it was not only a prerequisite for attendance on the BSO/SCTF postgraduate cranial course but also a factor among a number of other things for them to remain on the steering committee, especially considering the fluctuating standards of some of the non-GCRO osteopaths. Such an idea found some resonance with a number of American colleagues. In fairness too, like many others, Woodhead and Pascoe were unaware that Bingham, Langer, Armitstead and Fielding were endeavouring to shore up the profession's delicate unity under a degree of secrecy.[26]

Others on the committee made it clear that they supported attendance of non-GCRO members onto courses not necessarily located at the BSO. The BSO's very existence was looking more and more tenuous by the day. In time Pascoe and Woodhead resigned from the steering committee despite finding some sympathetic support among SCTF colleagues. It was declared:

"With respect to the changing political scene in the UK, we again fall back on our original purpose and goals. There would be a definite problem with accepting unqualified (non-GCRO) participants in a SCTF sponsored course".[27]

The message emanating from the Osteopathic Genesis Foundation, the Ministry of Health, and the King's Fund Committee on Statutory Regulation for Osteopaths was that unless the profession was united, no political progress could be made. Indeed, many of the non-GCRO osteopaths felt excluded from mainstream developments. It was Sir Tom Bingham, Jane Langer and Simon Fielding who went out of their way to include them at the very centre of discussion. Unfortunately, apart from Irwin Korr, no one in America was privy to these talks or negotiations. Even their British colleagues did not have all the information available that would have adequately explained the situation.[28]

The formidable Edna Lay, a senior member of the SCTF, could not quite substantiate her growing anger towards Dove, either. The following announcement in the January 1993 issue of the *Journal of Osteopathic Education* published by the GCRO clearly demonstrates her ire:

Osteopathy in the Cranial Field

16–21 April 1993 (5-day basic course). Venue: BCNO, Frazer House, 6 Netherhall Gardens, London NW3 5RR. Cost: tba. *Open to all osteopaths* [my italics]. For further information contact: The Registrar, The British Sutherland Cranial Faculty, 70 Belmont Road, Hereford HR2 7JW. Tel: 0432 356655.

Lay could not come to terms with UK government policy that only a unified osteopathic profession would be considered for statutory regulation. Nor had she been party to Rollin Becker's and John Harakal's verbal agreements with Dove. It was unfortunate that an elder colleague could not understand that no verbal agreement had been broken with this notice. All osteopaths including GCRO members had to take some sort of examination for inclusion on the General Osteopathic Council (GOsC). The Sutherland Cranial Faculty's invitation to all osteopaths was in the spirit of the times and one that was totally understood by the magnificent judge, Bingham. Dove's position had never changed. He had from the early 1970s been bridge building consistently with other groups and had included those groups onto the SCTF/BSO postgraduate courses that were negotiating entry to GCRO membership. He wrote numerous letters to John Harakal outlining UK osteopathy and its different associations. It was not his fault that the immediacy of serious illness afflicting Becker and Harakal should project the good-natured but inexperienced Michael Burruano into the hot seat of the SCTF presidency.[29]

Burruano could not possibly have known about the complexities of the arrangements that had been built on mutual trust. He was caught between an aggrieved Dove and an adamantly rebuking Edna. Matters were complicated further by British colleagues making the SCTF/BSO postgraduate course open to GCRO members only in contrast to the British Sutherland Cranial Faculty's basic course that could be attended by any osteopath. Burruano constantly reminded colleagues both sides of the Atlantic that the SCTF was a training institution, not a political one. He tried to dissuade Dove from resigning as an Associate SCTF Director, suggesting that his dissatisfaction merely stemmed from a private matter between him and Edna.[30] In fact, the landscape of British osteopathy was changing vastly and rapidly and Burruano had to deal with two British sponsored SCTF groups at odds with one another. It was not an unusual precedent historically. Jacques Duval, Colin Dove, Martin Pascoe and others had links with American counterparts but this was not a totally BSO inspired predicament.

Other UK schools played a crucial role in promoting the cranial concept and the European School of Osteopathy (ESO) was heavily involved in the development of cranial osteopathy. It held the first UK undergraduate cranial courses, followed later by the BSO, BCNO and other colleges. Susan Turner became an integral member of the British group. She was the first ESO graduate on the BSO postgraduate faculty and fostered special transatlantic contacts with Anne Wales, Michael Burruano and Frank Willard.[31] She spent many years running the ESO children's clinic, and is still much in demand as a postgraduate tutor and lecturer. Her ESO colleague, Thomas Attlee, continues to run his own postgraduate cranial establishment. His institute is one among a number of associations and establishments that have emerged since those pioneering days. Perhaps the most formidable has been the Osteopathic Children's Clinic (OCC) founded and led by the charismatic Stuart Korth.

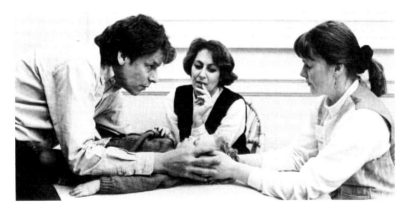

Fig. 30: Stuart Korth

Analysis

Sutherland developed ideas fairly similar to previous active therapies of phrenology and magnetic healing that were flourishing in the nineteenth century. By 1961, the US osteopathic medical schools had met the standards of regular medical schools and in consequence, the majority of osteopathic physicians and surgeons no longer practised manipulative therapy. Still's concepts remained central to traditional practitioners who declined rapidly in number but fought to uphold his values. Meanwhile, Sutherland's treatise became a clarion call to an even smaller but purposeful group of osteopathic physicians. Cranial osteopathy developed in the UK from US-trained osteopaths such as Emilie Jackson in the UK and determined practitioners from America who had been prepared to spread Sutherland's hypothesis to their colleagues in Paris and London fifty years or more ago. Additionally, Eddie Gilhooley, Denis Brookes, John Dixon and 'Sam' Grierson Currie disseminated Sutherland's work to British and French osteopathic students and contemporaries.

These two incongruent groups coalesced in a series of postgraduate courses in Europe and America: Jacques Duval, Colin Dove and Martin Pascoe on one side and Rollin Becker and John Harakal, under the auspices of the Sutherland Cranial Teaching Foundation (SCTF), on the other. Dove became a UK link between Becker and Harakal. For many years, the BSO postgraduate faculty held annual courses sponsored by SCTF, American speakers providing a major contribution. Cordial relations developed into transatlantic friendships, something that had been unrealized for 70 years. Dove assisted graduates from the ESO and the BCNO in joining theses courses (a SCTF prerequisite) prior to their entry on the GCRO.

Becker and Harakal were aware that ESO and BCNO graduates would be welcomed on these courses, preceding their GCRO membership under a gentleman's agreement. However, this lead to American dismay during a Brussels' SCTF course when some BCNO graduates attended without GCRO equivalent registration. In response, the AOA, the AAO and the Cranial Academy decreed attendance of all their courses must be restricted to US-trained osteopathic physicians in America. The SCTF was able to sponsor courses outside America for doctors, dentists and GCRO comparable osteopaths. Meanwhile, Anglo–American contacts, growing immeasurably stronger over the years, developed into friendships and study groups not bounded by AOA pronouncements to the otherwise.

In the UK, Dove was the architect of ESO entry to the GCRO, followed by BCNO inclusion. Cranial training became part of the school undergraduate curricula, firstly at the ESO and later at all colleges. Postgraduate courses were popular. From being a small insignificant number on the fringes, cranial osteopathy developed into a vibrant, even romantic, dynamic discipline. It no longer sought neither the blessing of its American counterparts nor found derision among some UK musculoskeletal protagonists. It came of age at a time when many colleagues felt constrained within a minor orthopaedic straitjacket. It now has two tasks to perform: a comprehensive rationale of how it works and the institution of small but well-structured clinical trials.

References

1. Fuller, R.C., *Mesmerism and the American Cure of Souls*. Philadelphia: University of Pennsylvania Press. 1982. p.132.
2. Ibid, pp.144–5.
3. Waddell, G., *The Back Pain Revolution*. Edinburgh: Churchill Livingstone. 2004. pp.268–9.
4. Gevitz, N., 'Osteopathic Medicine: from deviance to difference.' Edited by N. Gevitz. *Other Healers: Unorthodox Medicine in America*. Baltimore: John Hopkins University Press. 1988. p.128.
5. Fuller, *Mesmerism and the American Cure of Souls*. pp.138–9.
6. Gevitz, Osteopathic Medicine: From Deviance to Difference. p.128.
7. NOA Cranial Volumes: 1–4; code CRA/Files: 1–4.
8. Lowe, Ken, NOA DVD Interview 2011.
9. Dove C.I., NOA DVD 3 Cranial Interview 2008.
10. Pascoe, M., Correspondence: 27th May 2011.
11. Dove C.I., NOA Colin Dove Collection Cranial Correspondence 1980–2005 Vol.4. Cranial Osteopathy in Great Britain: Cranial letter/Winter 1988. p.1.
12. Dove C.I., NOA DVD 3 Cranial Interview. 2008.
13. Dove, Cranial Osteopathy in Great Britain: Cranial letter/Winter 1988. p.1.
14. Ibid.
15. Dove C.I., NOA DVD 3 Cranial Interview. 2008.
16. Dove, Cranial Osteopathy in Great Britain: Cranial letter/Winter 1988. p.2.
17. Jealous J., NOA Colin Dove Collection Cranial Correspondence 1980–2005 Vol. 4 Letter to CI Dove p.2.
18. Harakal J., NOA Colin Dove Collection Cranial Correspondence 1980–2005 Vol. 4 Letter to CI Dove 12.10.1984.
19. Dove C.I., NOA Colin Dove Collection Cranial Correspondence 1980–2005 Vol. 4 Letter to J Harakal 5.01.1985.
20. Harakal J., NOA Colin Dove Collection Cranial Correspondence 1980–2005 Vol. 4 letter to CI Dove 18.9.1985.
21. Dove, Cranial Osteopathy in Great Britain: Cranial letter/Winter 1988. p.2.
22. Turner Susan, NOA DVD Interview 2008.

23. Dove C.I., NOA Colin Dove Collection Cranial Correspondence 1980–2005 Vol. 4 Letter to Michael Burruano 9.10.1992. p.1.
24. Turner S.
25. Handoll N. NOA DVD Interview 2010.
26. Woodhead, N., Conversation 31st May 2011.
27. Burruano M., NOA Colin Dove Collection Cranial Correspondence 1980–2005 Vol. 4 Letter to CI Dove 19.10.1992. p.1.
28. Turner S.
29. Lay, E. NOA Colin Dove Collection Cranial Correspondence 1980–2005 Vol. 4 Letter to CI Dove 23-8-1995.
30. Burruano M. NOA Colin Dove Collection Cranial Correspondence 1980–2005 Vol. 4 Letter to CI Dove 20-6-1995.
31. Turner S.

Chapter 11

Osteopathy in Britain: Past and Future

Précis

Osteopathy has been hampered by a tradition of discouraging debate and healthy discussion. Inheriting tenets and principles and ALSO clinical procedures based on subjective skills, palpation and observation have disadvantaged students. Part of the blame lies with professional disunity among the numerous disparate factions. Within the confines of a more united profession, how can we develop more open and frank debate without personal rancour dominating the debate? Osteopathy has already jumped many difficult hurdles on its way to becoming the profession it is today in Britain. But at what price has this been achieved? It could be argued that its overriding philosophical principles have vanished. We have to return to those rambling, Littlejohn discourses to understand why AT Still found this remarkable, physically slight academic such a threat to his position. Littlejohn's ideas on adjustment and adaption of the human condition has particular resonance today. If we can change our school curricula to acknowledge Littlejohn's original tenets, the profession will be set on a more fruitful path.

Concluding Analysis

AT Still's ideas interpreted initially by Bill Smith explained osteopathy as a panacea of all ills. This lightning bonesetter proposed that where a bone was out of place a dysfunction developed. It was thought that mechanical malfunction resulted in disturbed bodily function, impacting on the brain and spiritual nature of the person. Smith was given the impossible task of describing and discerning Still's philosophies. Still kept much of his past disguised. His language was flowery and akin to that of a preacher. Although Still was an astute clinician, his academic knowledge was fragmentary. His anatomical terminology and detail had little bearing on its Latin and Greek origins, which made him a rather vague and incomplete anatomy lecturer and demonstrator. It is clear why he needed to secure Smith's help in teaching the subject in the very early days of the American School of Osteopathy (ASO) in Kirksville, Missouri. The pioneering ASO students had great difficulty in following his manipulative sessions too.

Although Still's public persona as a medically reforming Abraham Lincoln served a missionary purpose, Bill Smith's presence legitimised osteopathy in the face of medical opposition. Still appeared to rejoice in a mid-Western life devoid of urban culture and one that possessed only vestigial healthcare, social life and education. He loved to harness simple basic mechanical ideas and homespun philosophy to osteopathy, rendering it easily understood by Kirksville folk and those from surrounding communities. Initially many were suspicious of his claims but these feelings were shelved when his reputation brought visitors and economic benefits to the town. Still's standing and practice expanded rapidly, dependent upon his charismatic status. Smith's attention was directed towards evolving the ASO course despite Still's obstinacy. Still's insightful creed resonated with a number of people, from those who were suffering from physical pain to others keen to train as osteopaths. (Both groups incidentally added large financial sums to the Still family coffers.) From this tradition emerged a belief system based on unsubstantive doctrines and largely unquestioned loyalty to Still's provenance and leadership.

In 1898, the three Littlejohn brothers joined Bill Smith on the ASO faculty, only for them to be removed at a stroke by Still two years later. The move was done under the guise of protestations from other faculty members who were resisting further academic improvements, and the Littlejohn/Smith axis that was apparently disdainful of other, less educated, faculty. Whether this was a set-up or not, Smith et al would have steered a more open approach towards osteopathic education at Kirksville. The Littlejohn brothers were permitted to finish their courses but the Still family continued to pursue a kind of vendetta against JM Littlejohn. It established a tradition of intolerance to other like-minded people and an unhealthy disregard for the motives of those who questioned Still's tenets and principles.

In due course, American Osteopathic Association (AOA) associated schools were inspected by Abraham Flexner for his report on North American medical schools (1910). Flexner's highly critical censure of osteopathic education was essentially ignored. His report on eight osteopathic schools came under the chapter heading 'sectarian'. He stated that they should emulate their orthodox counterparts and upgrade the education they offered. He commented that clinical diagnostic standards should be the same across the board whether the practitioner was osteopathic or medical, regardless that the treatments offered would differ widely.[1] He found osteopathic students' entry qualifications to be very basic and rudimentary; many of them had come from small towns or farming stock. Flexner's report severely criticised the low level osteopathic college entrant requirements as well as poor laboratory access and clinical training, especially during in-house hospital training.

Flexner's recommendations were adopted by the American Medical Association (AMA) with some impetus from public interest but implementation took 25 years to complete and as a result of the process, 60% of closed. His resolution that all medical schools should be run by an independent board of trustees rather than having their ownership placed into the hands of individuals was instigated in some osteopathic colleges including Littlejohn's in Chicago. The changes deprived JM Littlejohn of his position as head of the school and fuelled his return to Britain, away from mainstream osteopathy. Flexner reforms were set aside by the AOA for another 25 years, while a more fundamentalist, evangelical movement thrived; chiropractic had prevented the profession from returning to an earlier appreciation of its roots. Still's death in 1917 opened the door for change.

The AOA board of trustees duly made various pronouncements to upgrade entry requirements and course improvements but it was not until the mid-1930s that its colleges implemented many of them.[2] It was a cohort of reforming osteopaths who took on their majority traditional colleagues by exhorting an evolutionary pathway towards orthodoxy.[3] Their role was facilitated by the profession's apparent inability to gain full practice rights akin to those held by MDs and traditionalists who faced competition from chiropractic. One survey by two Canadian academicians compared the quality of osteopathic schools with three medical ones. They concluded that osteopathic graduates failed to achieve standards equal to those of medical graduates and therefore should not be ascribed the title, "Physician and Surgeon".[4]

The AMA duress emphasised the importance of this report to all state legislature boards. It stressed the disparity between the two graduate groups. Something had to be done to amend the inequality. As a result, the AOA associated colleges appointed LE Blauch, an educational consultant who had recently conducted a Flexner-type survey of North American dental schools. John E Rogers, Chairman of the AOA Bureau of Professional Education, accompanied Blauch while he collated data and analysed his findings from the osteopathic schools. Much to the dismay of the profession, his conclusions were similar to those of the previous Canadian report. Consequently, the osteopathic schools did embark on a root and branch reform but it took 25 years to complete[5] and osteopaths were forced to pursue the orthodox path taken over two decades before by the AMA.

It is necessary to consider what all this has to do with UK osteopathy. During the early years of the twentieth century and through the Second World War less than 100 graduates from the AOA affiliated colleges came to the UK. A smaller number of graduates from non-affiliated colleges, mainly from the New Jersey School, New York, settled in Britain.[6] These two groups comprised of traditional osteopaths who adhered very much to the profession's original tenets and precepts despite the ever-growing reforming cohort. Traditionalist numbers dwindled in America and no further graduates appear to have settled in Britain after 1945. Although US-trained practitioners made a sizable number of osteopaths, many never joined the General Council and Register of Osteopaths (GCRO), which became a BSO graduate institution within four years of inception. British Osteopathic Association (BOA) hostility continued to abate against the Osteopathic Association of Great Britain (OAGB) BSO graduates. Ironically, it was Littlejohn's BSO which emerged in post-war Britain as the most influential school.

In 1948, following JM Littlejohn's death, the new principle Shilton Webster-Jones (Webber) took the BSO not only on a narrowly defined course to train students within the confines of biophysical medicine but he also handpicked certain people to assist him in this task. Webber was exasperated by the energy-sapping behaviour of particular individuals who behaved like gurus. These people rallied some sympathetically minded individuals into scattered pockets of dissension, much to the pleasure of UK osteopathy's many enemies. Be that as it may, these five individuals, Webber, Clem Middleton, Audrey Smith, Margot Gore and later Colin Dove, formed a group willing to work tirelessly to improve training standards.[7]

The BSO faculty faced severe opposition and personal denigration from other groups, which furthered the profession's inability to discuss things healthily without rancour. The BSO core curriculum was adopted by all schools joining the GCRO and continued to set educational standards for all colleges within the General Osteopathic Council (GOsC). Even though some discussion took place, it was inevitably fairly superficial and intermittent. It was left to Kim Burton and Jon Thompson, co-editors of the *British Osteopathic Journal*, to question and address the quality of subject matter in its published papers.

The journal was later replaced by *Clinical Biomechanics*, published partly in response to the scarcity of authentic osteopathic articles and ever-increasing contributions from experts outside the profession. At the same time cranial therapy became a cause célèbre for those who appeared to doubt the simplistic biophysical concept of osteopathy but also baulked at the loss of the artistic side of osteopathic practice in the face of greater scientific input. Some dialogue did take place between the protagonists but pivotal to the cranial cognoscenti was whether one could 'feel' three dimensionally or spatially. According to cranial practitioners, on this ability it was fundamental to build layers of palpatory experiential knowledge. Instead of discussing separate ends of the osteopathic spectrum, biomechanical and cranial practice, true to form, personal denigration became the modus operandi and detracted from any sensible dialogue. Without a tradition for healthy debate, students and practitioners have found it difficult to enter into any extended discussion of contentious subjects without resorting to personal rancour and disrespect coming to the fore.

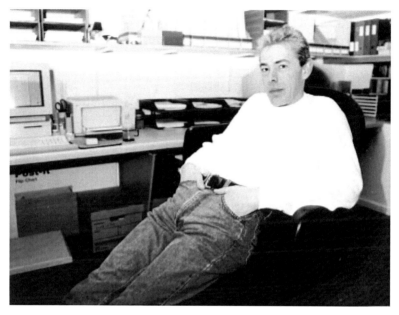

Fig. 31: Kim Burton

If some of Kim Burton's detractors had listened more intently to his ideas they might have realised that not only was his work on spinal flexibility worth reading but also his mind had remained flexible too. Ironically, his co-research work on a biopsychosocial model opens up possibilities for determining an understanding of cranial therapy. Somehow we must break this unhealthy tradition of personal invective, which has been so prominent within osteopathic history. Osteopathic tenets and principles are not sacred testaments but important topics for each osteopathic generation to question, discuss and re-interpret in an open, generous, healthy atmosphere. For this, one school needs to start a revolutionary change by reigniting a pioneering spirit of open-minded discourse, an ethos quite alien to our historical roots.

Perhaps we have to embrace technology more, especially that which would rid us of so much paperwork. For example, case history taking is one of those essential disciplines that lends itself to software innovation via laptops and iPads. Why cannot red and yellow flag clinical considerations be factored into such programmes? We must start building up syndrome clusters in our practices to acknowledge specific outcomes based on a more specific triage development, bringing in psychosocial factors as well. Jo Wildy in her usual inimitable, cogent style sets out a hypothesis to restore some sort of balance between the cerebral hemispheres interpretation, which in modern life are out of kilter. As Iain McGilchrist describes in his book *The Master and his Emissary: the divided brain and the making of the western world*, "the left and right hemispheres co-exist together on a daily basis but have a fundamentally different set of values and priorities".

It is the left side of the brain that dominates our life according to Wildy and McGilchrist, "an increasingly mechanistic, fragmented, decontextualized world, marked by unwarranted optimism mixed with paranoia and a feeling of emptiness has come about due to the unopposed action of a dysfunctional left hemisphere". We now know what Wildy means by being right-minded, she being right hemisphere dominant and an advocate of experiential knowledge and 'non-verbal communication'. What is magnificent about her paper is its scholarship, style and cognisance. One might not agree with her conclusions but one defends its freshness, rationale and importance within the debate. She postulates a need to clearly define our distinctiveness and perhaps our uniqueness based on our tenets and principles, to expound a more inclusive and unified profession and reform our UK schools so that they provide more wide-ranging courses similar to Continental European curricula.[8] It appears that by considering such issues the profession can agree to changes in school curricula.

Perhaps we should focus on understanding what disciplines may be involved in different syndromes and from this, consider changing and amending such subjects. If it is suggested by right hemisphere dominant quarters that they cannot explain what is happening in therapy, it is best to inform them with respect that this is not good enough, but the dialogue should ensue. This ethos must resonate throughout our schools. Their curricula and courses should be more open so that students are able to contemplate their subjective skills such as palpation and observation as incomplete clinical references rather than abilities that can refine to almost proficient levels of excellence, bordering on mystical comprehension. This idea may be at the heart of what many right hemisphere dominant people believe but it offers little help in advancing our understanding, nor does explain their interpretations of health and dysfunction. Both these attributes, palpation and observation, can be useful in assisting in clinical examination and treatment but only in the context and awareness of their limitations.

Arguably, students should be allowed to reassess their commitment to graduate as musculoskeletal practitioners only. Osteopathic education could be revised to support this and provoke more thought. Schools should think about compressing courses into a three-year full-time BSc without a dissertation but one that did feature clinical training, had an emphasis on psychosocial matters, the complexity of pain and included final and clinical competence exams. This would make the final year more eventful for students and enable them to choose from a wide selection of disciplines.

A new one year MSc course could include an expanded dissertation, psychology and CBT, occupational medicine, ergonomics, musculoskeletal medicine, community medicine, health and safety and cranial and other osteopathic specialisms. It could be taught over three evenings a week in a two-semester continual assessment programme that would involve lectures and tutorials. Some of the topics would embrace the whole cohort, while others could be specific to the modality undertaken. The dissertation would require greater cognition and commitment, taking students out of their 'comfort zone' and comprise of 45% of the total marks. Supervisors and referees would be academic staff proficient to examine at this level. Of course, these timetables would have to be amended for those using distance-learning and extended-learning pathways. Introducing innovation into our approach could lead to a greater exchange of ideas and free the profession from the straitjacket of minor orthopaedics.

As Professor Stephen Tyreman says, these are exciting times for osteopathy. I would like to offer a plea to step back and more realistically reassess our contribution to health. Historically, there has always been a yearning to return to a golden age, which, quite frankly, never existed. Moreover, misconceptions abound to deflect any serious reappraisal. Although most clinical faculties exist within the same complex, in reality they appear to be a distance apart, countenancing 'them and us' notions.

Dedicated clinical staff need to be included in the reassessment and their worth appreciated, not only in changing direction but also in realising the need to do so. Any discerning student keeps their views to their friends, struggling to balance a wide disparity between academia, osteopathic subjects and clinical studies. Even the final clinical exams affirm a clinical ritual which may be considerably irrelevant and unsuitable for purpose. Therefore, the aim should be to entice students to use their brains rather than rely on well-intended subjective unsubstantive data, which is confusing, dogmatic and, perhaps misdirected. The time seems right now to discuss change.

The strategy of osteopathic clinical treatment should be to construct a working hypothesis from presenting symptoms based on a triage system of clinical examination using more general subjective observation and palpation skills (rather than being over-concerned with specific palpatory and musculoskeletal nuances) whilst also identifying underlying dysfunction. First and foremost we must attend to the presenting symptoms; to encourage; retrain aspects of patient routines that maintain these dysfunctional behaviours by setting aside time to address these, whilst using an assortment of psychological, sociological and musculoskeletal skills to help the patient understand pain, discomfort and unease in a physical framework; and finally developing self-sufficiency, within a mutually acknowledged timescale.

Constructing techniques in rhythmical, soothing and deep relaxatory approaches rather than more aggressive or disruptive, anxiety-making techniques would be advisable. A palpatory dimension would give reassurance and emotional/physical protection during treatment. We should impose a limit of perhaps six sessions maximum (although this should not be written in stone).

My hypothesis supports a notion that a patient's presenting symptoms are not necessarily their real reason for attending but a subconscious desire for patients to seek practitioners to determine what the underlying dysfunction might be. Far more psychological/sociological expertise in training is required to discover underlying problems, while at the same time the presenting symptoms must be addressed. It may be that case history taking continues over 2–3 sessions or more. It would be part of a dialogue which places much on what is revealed and patient cooperation during the process. Using a triage system, can one identify any pathology or urgent neurological condition requiring urgent medical intervention? What of pain? How much 'illness behaviour' dominates the patient? Can you start to identify underlying dysfunction?

Overlying this appraisal would be a more general understanding of subjective observation and palpation without their specificity, subsequently noting any gross observable physical feature from a general perspective at a little distance. Palpation should be gentle, non-specific and more to do with reassurance and handling the patient during essential orthopaedic, neurological and other tests. Once triage has underpinned a patient's symptoms, it should determine a reasonable working diagnosis and prognosis of symptoms whilst the underlying dysfunction addressed and subsidiary factors considered but in an informal way. Part of the relationship between patient/practitioner is building up trust, allowing the patient to be reassured within a safe environment but as part of the decision-making process.

In a sense I have come full circle. One of my major themes was to consider AT Still's troublesome time from 1898 to 1900, the period when the three Littlejohn brothers attended Kirksville. Clearly, Still was alarmed at JM Littlejohn's capacity to take his own (partially borrowed) ideas and expand upon them in ways that he found so threatening. Here was an academic who appeared to be taking over his very own creation with enormous industry and output. That JM Littlejohn should languish the best part of four decades in exile, so to speak, away from mainstream American osteopathy, is a great loss. It is probable that he would have sought a third way to evolve osteopathy, not returning to its traditional roots but competing against a vibrant chiropractic profession. He would not have taken the orthodox route mimicking the medical profession but instead followed a biopsychosocial methodology whereby dysfunction within these categories would have been assessed. JM Littlejohn's discourses have recently undergone critical scrutiny[9] and it is hoped that his contribution and rehabilitation will provide us with a renovated compass to navigate these interesting times. Central to this premise is the need to understand an individual's ability to adjust and adapt to change. In this way, we have gone full circle back to Quimby and AT Still.

References

1.   Flexner, A. *Medical Education in the United States and Canada: a report to the Carnegie Foundation for the advancement of teaching.* The Merrymount Press: Boston, 1910 p.164.

2.   Gevitz, N., *The DOs: Osteopathic Medicine in America.* John Hopkins University Press. 1982. p.79.

3.   BMA. Quality of Osteopathic Education in the USA. BMA Committee on Osteopathy Part 4, no. Ost 16. 1.2.1935. p.1–3.

4.   Gevitz, N. *The DOs.* p.83.

5.   Ibid.

6.   NOA GCRO Council minutes 12.3.1937. pp.77–8, 80, 82.

7.   Dove C.I. NOA DVD interview Volume 1 –The Early Years. 2007.

8.   Wildy, J., The brain, the mind and the osteopath. *Osteopathy Today.* April 2011. 17(3): pp.12–15; 21–3.

9.   Tyreman S. Philosophical Writings of J Martin Littlejohn. Osteopathic History Group 4th symposium June 2011 DVD disc 1.

Index